Simplified
Diet Manual

Simplified
Diet Manual

Tenth Edition

Iowa Dietetic Association

Edited by Andrea K. Maher, R.D., L.D.

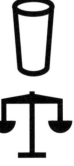

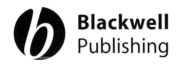
Blackwell
Publishing

Editor: Andrea K. Maher, R.D., L.D. serves as clinical dietitian for Select Specialty Hospital of the Quad Cities, Davenport, Iowa, the first long-term acute care hospital in Iowa, and as consultant dietitian for Eagle Point Nursing and Rehab, Clinton, Iowa, a 114 bed facility including a dementia unit and skilled care.

Reviewers: Jane Linnenbrink, RD, LD; Char Kooima, RD, LD, CDE; Kathleen Niedert, MBA, RD, LD, FADA; Brenda Brink, RD, LD; Jane Reinhart-Martin RD, LD; Jody Kealey, RD, LD; Heather Illig, RD, LD; Carol Hill, RD, LD; Cheryl Stimson, MS, RD, LD; Marti Bradbury, RD, LD; Susan Boardsen, MPH, RD, LD; Wendy Brewer, RD, LD; Deb Hassebrock, RD, LD; Rose Hoenig, RD, LD; Jan Steffen, RD, LD; Kay Wing, RD, LD, CDE; Chris Timmons, RD, LD; Beverlee Clearman, RD, LD; Hayley Kouba, RD, LD; and Roxane Patton, RD, LD.

Blackwell Publishing Professional
2121 State Avenue, Ames, Iowa 50014, USA

Orders: 1-800-862-6657
Office: 1-515-292-0140
Fax: 1-515-292-3348
Web site: www.blackwellprofessional.com

Blackwell Publishing Ltd
9600 Garsington Road, Oxford OX4 2DQ, UK
Tel.: +44 (0)1865 776868

Blackwell Publishing Asia
550 Swanston Street, Carlton, Victoria   3053,
Australia
Tel.: +61 (0)3 8359 1011

Authorization to photocopy items for internal or personal use, or the internal or personal use of specific clients, is granted by Blackwell Publishing, provided that the base fee is paid directly to the Copyright Clearance Center, 222 Rosewood Drive, Danvers, MA 01923. For those organizations that have been granted a photocopy license by CCC, a separate system of payments has been arranged. The fee code for users of the Transactional Reporting Service is ISBN-13: 978-0-8138-1878-8/2007.

The Iowa Dietetic Association acknowledges the use of the following registered trademarks: Malt-O-Meal, Resource, Boost Breeze, Enlive, NuBasics, Chex Mix, Townhouse, Ritz, Doritos, Goldfish crackers, Oreo, Honey Maid, Starburst, Lifesavers, Rice Krispies, Cream of Rice, Cream of Wheat, Kool-Aid, Tang, Country Time Lemonade, Accent, Lactaid, Dairy Ease, Montina, Ovaltine, Postum, Benecol, Take Control.

Printed and bound in United States of America by Sheridan Books, Inc.

First edition, ©1958 Iowa State University Press
Second edition, ©1961 Iowa State University Press
Third edition, ©1969 Iowa State University Press
Fourth edition, ©1975 Iowa State University Press
Fifth edition, ©1984 Iowa State University Press
Sixth edition, ©1990 Iowa State University Press
Seventh edition, ©1995 Iowa State University Press
Eighth edition, ©1999 Iowa State University Press
Ninth edition, ©2002 Iowa State Press
Tenth edition, ©2007 Blackwell Publishing

Library of Congress Cataloging-in-Publication Data

Simplified diet manual/edited by Andrea K. Maher; Iowa Dietetic
   Association.–10th ed.
      p. ; cm.
   Includes bibliographical references and index.
   ISBN-13: 978-0-8138-1878-8 (alk. paper)
   ISBN-10: 0-8138-1878-8 (alk. paper)
   1. Diet therapy. 2. Menus. 3. Recipes. I. Maher, Andrea K.
   II. Iowa Dietetic Association.
     [DNLM: 1. Diet Therapy. 2. Dietary Services. 3. Dietetics
   –methods. 4. Menu Planning. WB 400 S612 2007]
RM216.R63 2007
613.2–dc22
                                                          2006018853

The last digit is the print number: 9 8 7 6 5

Contents

Appendixes   151

About the Book

The tenth edition of the *Simplified Diet Manual* marks 54 years of its publication by the Iowa Dietetic Association. In 1953 Nina Kagarice Bigsby, the dietary consultant to small hospitals and nursing homes for the Iowa State Department of Health, began a survey of diets that were being prescribed by physicians in Iowa. A trial manual was compiled, used for several months in ten Iowa hospitals, and evaluated by a special committee of the Iowa Dietetic Association; then a manuscript was prepared for publication.

Hospitals and long-term care facilities in every state and many foreign countries now use the *Simplified Diet Manual*. The Iowa Dietetic Association receives the royalties from its publication and uses them for the organization's mission: "Leading the future of dietetics."

Through the ten editions, many thoughtful, practical, and insightful dietitians have contributed their expertise, ideas, and experience to keep the *Simplified Diet Manual* up-to-date while retaining its straightforward and uncomplicated style.

References cited within the text can be found in the Resource section at the end of the book. Cited materials are numbered to correlate with their source.

Study guide questions have been incorporated within the diet manual to give practice in applying the information. The material included has been carefully selected to cover basic information on the General Diet and its modifications for individually prescribed diets. Successful completion of this study will improve the skill of foodservice employees.

1. Read and study each chapter of the *Simplified Diet Manual*.
2. Read the study guide questions that follow each chapter, fill in the blanks, and do the work requested. Refer back to the chapter as needed.
3. Look over the answers to make sure you have completed each question to the best of your knowledge. In some questions several answers are possible.
4. See Appendix 12 for the suggested responses; they may be removed from the book. If any of your answers are wrong, the instructor will discuss the correct answer with you. If the answer section is left in the book, students should complete each section

and then compare the answers with those in the answer section. The instructor should review items the students found difficult.

The tenth edition was edited by Andrea Maher, R.D., L.D., a consultant dietitian in long-term care. It reflects the comments and recommendations of Iowa Dietetic Association members and other users of this manual. These suggestions led to the revisions and additions that make this edition as comprehensive and useful as possible, consistent with current advances in Medical Nutrition Therapy.

The tenth edition was endorsed by the Iowa Dietetic Association Publications Committee, Anne Tabor, M.P.H., R.D., L.D., chair; the Iowa Dietetic Association Board, Sue Clarahan, R.D., L.D., President; the Iowa Department of Inspections and Appeals, Health Facilities Division, Judith A. Walrod, RD, LD, Elder Affairs; the Iowa Consulting Dietetians in Health Care Facilities, Char Kooima, R.D., L.D., CDE chair; and Debra D. Dawson, C.D.M., C.F.P.P., Iowa Dietary Managers Association Spokesperson.

The major changes in this edition are outlined in detail in the Preface.

PREFACE

In the early 1980s, the Iowa Dietetic Association adopted the policy of reviewing and revising its publications, including the *Simplified Diet Manual*, on a regular cycle. The tenth edition reflects the sixth time the manual has been revised under this policy. Regular review has kept the association alert to the dynamic nature of the field of nutrition.

The tenth edition of the *Simplified Diet Manual* strives to keep up with the changes in the science of nutrition and society trends, but retains its basic purpose. In a simplified manner it provides a guide for the prescription and interpretation of diets or nutrition plans.

Individuals' nutrition plans must meet their needs both physiologically and emotionally. Nutritional adequacy must be emphasized, but the consideration of both these needs will contribute to the greatest success. In all cases, we advocate the most liberal, least restrictive diets to meet nutritional needs, especially for residents in long-term care.

Several changes were made to this edition:

- Revision of the Guidelines for Diet Planning based on *Dietary Guidelines for Americans 2005* and USDA's MyPyramid
- Revision of Vitamin A foods listed in the "Outstanding" category
- Revision of Food For The Day tables based on MyPyramid
- Update on Meeting Nutritional Needs of Older People, referencing the American Dietetic Association's position: Liberalization of the Diet Prescription for Older Adults
- Inclusion of National Dysphagia Diet tables (2002, American Dietetic Association)
- Revision of the Diets for Weight Management chapter, emphasizing the importance of diet, exercise, and behavior modification
- Addition of the Bariatric/Gastric Bypass Diet
- Deletion of the Limited Concentrated Sweets Diet
- Revision of the Diets for Diabetes chapter
- Addition of the Modified Renal Diet
- Addition of the Fluid Restriction Guidelines
- Addition of Food Allergies and Intolerances
- Addition of the Phenylketonuria Diet
- Addition of Developmental Disabilities and Chronic Disease

- Update on the Dietary Reference Intakes to include all values released through 2004 (see Appendixes 1 through 4)
- Expanded Body Mass Index table to include category of extreme obesity
- Revision of Vitamin A, Vitamin C and Zinc Content of Selected Foods using the Agricultural Research Service Nutrient Database for Standard Reference, Release 18
- Inclusion of Calcium and Iron Content of Selected Foods (see Appendixes 8 and 10)
- Revision of Exchange Lists for Meal Planning (2003, American Dietetic Association)
- Inclusion of study guide questions at the end of each chapter for training foodservice employees in health care facilities that are served by a registered dietitian or dietary consultant.

The *Simplified Diet Manual* includes suggested meal patterns with most diets. As the use of the manual has spread, we realize that the names we use for meals do not always fit those used in other regions and countries. For meal planning purposes, we define meal names as follows:

> **Breakfast:** *The first meal of the day, served shortly after rising.*
> **Dinner:** *The largest meal of the day. It may be served either midday or in the evening, depending on local custom.*
> **Lunch or Supper:** *A lighter meal than dinner, it is served either at midday or evening. When served midday it is often called lunch, but if served at night, it is usually referred to as supper.*
> **Snack:** *A small amount of food offered in addition to main meals.*

Simplified
Diet Manual

CHAPTER 1

GUIDELINES FOR
Diet Planning

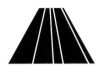

Adequate nourishment is essential to the maintenance of good health and to recovery from illness. As the body of nutrition research has grown, the recognition of the role of diet in the treatment and prevention of chronic diseases such as heart disease, diabetes, hypertension, and cancer has captured the attention of the medical community, the media, and the American public.

For example, at one time, the primary concern in treating diabetes was simply controlling blood sugars by monitoring the amount of carbohydrate people with diabetes consumed. Today, controlling body weight, blood pressure, and total saturated fat intake are considered important strategies in the treatment of diabetes to lower clients' risk of developing heart disease.

In the 1940s and 1950s, health concern focused on preventing nutritional deficiencies caused by lack of essential vitamins and minerals. Food guides were designed to prevent these deficiencies by recommending the number of servings Americans should eat from various food groups. In the first decade of the twenty-first century, attention has turned to the health consequences of consuming too much of some nutrients, especially sugar, fat, saturated fat, cholesterol, and sodium.

Current dietary recommendations for Americans are based on two complementary resources: the *Dietary Reference Intakes* (DRIs) and the *Dietary Guidelines for Americans*. The DRIs are published by the Food and Nutrition Board of the National Academy of Sciences. They are intended to be "reference values that are quantitative estimates of the nutrient intakes to be used for planning and assessing diets for healthy people." This edition of the *Simplified Diet Manual* includes the DRIs available to date (see Appendixes 1–4).

Dietary Guidelines for Americans

The *Dietary Guidelines for Americans 2005*, published by the U.S. Department of Agriculture and the U.S. Department of Health and Human Services, outlines a set of nine key messages for healthy Americans 2 years of age and older. These messages provide science-based advice to promote health and to reduce risk of major chronic diseases through diet and physical activity. The intent of the *Dietary Guidelines* is to summarize and synthesize knowledge regarding individual nutrients and food components into recommendations for a pattern of eating that can be adopted by the public. A basic premise of the *Dietary Guidelines* is that nutrient needs should be met primarily through consuming foods. Dietary supplements, while recommended in some cases, cannot replace a healthful diet. Key recommendations are grouped under nine inter-related focus areas:

- Consume a variety of foods within and among the basic food groups while staying within energy needs.
- Control calorie intake to manage body weight.
- Be physically active every day.
- Increase daily intake of fruits and vegetables, whole grains, and nonfat or low-fat milk and milk products.
- Choose fats wisely for good health.
- Choose carbohydrates wisely for good health.
- Choose and prepare foods with little salt.
- If you drink alcoholic beverages, do so in moderation.
- Keep food safe to eat.

MyPyramid

The U.S. Department of Agriculture (USDA) released the MyPyramid food guidance system in 2005, based on both the *Dietary Guidelines for Americans 2005* and the Dietary Reference Intakes from the National Academy of Sciences. The key tool of this guidance system is the website, www.mypyramid.gov. The new pyramid symbolizes a personalized approach to healthy eating and physical activity (see fig 1.1).

Using MyPyramid

The principles of the USDA MyPyramid food guidance system form the basis for the diets in this manual. The Food Guide Pyramid includes recommendations for the number of servings from each group daily; however, federal and state regulations for institutions may not

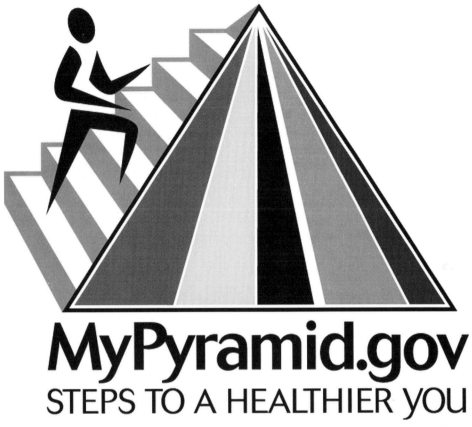

MyPyramid.gov
STEPS TO A HEALTHIER YOU

Figure 1.1. The MyPyramid food guidance system symbolizes a personalized approach to healthy eating and physical activity.

exactly match the recommendations. Menu planners must be knowledgeable of regulations affecting their facility.

Personalization

Personalization is shown by the person on the steps, the different calorie levels listed on the website, and the slogan. Find the kinds and amounts of food to eat each day at www.mypyramid.gov.

Gradual Improvement

Gradual improvement is encouraged by the slogan "Steps to a Healthier You." It suggests that individuals can benefit from taking small steps to improve their diet and lifestyle each day.

Physical Activity

Activity is represented by the steps and the person climbing them, as a reminder of the importance of daily physical activity.

Variety

Variety is symbolized by the 6 color bands representing the five food groups of MyPyramid and oils. Foods from all groups are needed each day for good health.

Moderation

Moderation is represented by the narrowing of each food group from bottom to top. The wider base stands for foods with little or no solid fats or added sugars. These should be selected more often. The narrower top area stands for foods containing more added sugars and solid fats.

Proportionality

Proportionality is shown by the different widths of the food group bands. The widths suggest how much food a person should choose from each group. The widths are a general guide, not exact proportions. Check the website for the amount that is right for each person.

How Much Is Needed?

The MyPyramid tables show suggested amounts of food to consume from the basic food groups, subgroups, and oils to meet recommended nutrient intakes at 12 different calorie levels. Nutrient and energy contributions from each group are calculated according to the nutrient-dense forms of foods in each group (i.e., lean meats and fat-free milk). The tables also show the discretionary calorie allowance that can be accommodated within each calorie level, in addition to the suggested amounts of nutrient-dense forms of foods in each group.

What Counts as a Serving?

▪ GRAINS GROUP: 3–10 OUNCE EQUIVALENTS DAILY

The Grains Group includes any food made from wheat, rice, oats, cornmeal, barley, or another cereal grain. Bread, pasta, oatmeal, breakfast cereals, tortillas, and grits are examples.

Grains are divided into two subgroups: whole grains and refined grains. Whole grains contain the entire grain kernel—the bran, germ, and endosperm. Examples include:

- Whole-wheat flour
- Bulgur (cracked wheat)
- Oatmeal
- Whole cornmeal
- Brown rice

FOOD INTAKE PATTERNS

Daily Amount of Food from Each Group

Calorie Level	1,000	1,200	1,400	1,600	1,800	2,000	2,200	2,400	2,600	2,800	3,000	3,200
Fruits (cups)	1	1	1.5	1.5	1.5	2	2	2	2	2.5	2.5	2.5
Vegetables (cups)	1	1.5	1.5	2	2.5	2.5	3	3	3.5	3.5	4	4
Grains (ounce equivalents)	3	4	5	5	6	6	7	8	9	10	10	10
Meat and Beans (ounce equivalents)	2	3	4	5	5	5.5	6	6.5	6.5	7	7	7
Milk (cups)	2	2	2	3	3	3	3	3	3	3	3	3
Oils/Fat (tsp)	3	4	4	5	5	6	6	7	8	8	10	11
Discretionary Calorie Allowance	165	171	171	132	195	267	290	362	410	426	512	648

Refined grains have been milled, a process that removes the bran and germ. This is done to give grains a finer texture and improve their shelf life, but it also removes dietary fiber, iron, and many B vitamins. Some examples of refined grain products are:

- White flour
- Degermed cornmeal
- White bread
- White rice

Most refined grains are *enriched*. This means certain B vitamins (thiamin, riboflavin, niacin, folic acid) and iron are added back after processing. Fiber is not added back to enriched grains. Check the ingredient list on refined grain products to make sure that the word "enriched" is included in the grain name.

The Grains Group provides many nutrients, including dietary fiber, several B vitamins (thiamin, riboflavin, niacin, and folate), and minerals (iron, magnesium, and selenium). Consuming foods rich in fiber, such as whole grains, as part of a healthy diet reduces the risk of coronary heart disease and may reduce constipation. Eating at least three ounce-equivalents a day of whole grains may help with weight management. At least half of all grains consumed should be whole grains.

COUNT AS 1 OUNCE EQUIVALENT:
1 slice of bread
½ cup of cooked rice, cooked pasta, or cooked cereal
1 cup ready-to-eat cereal

■ VEGETABLE GROUP: 1–4 CUPS DAILY

The Vegetable Group includes any vegetable or 100% vegetable juice. They may be raw or cooked; fresh, frozen, canned, or dried/dehydrated; and may be whole, cut-up, or mashed.

VEGETABLE SUBGROUPS (Cups per Week)						
Calorie Level	1,000	1,200	1,400	1,600	1,800	2,000
Dark Green	1	1.5	1.5	2	3	3
Orange	0.5	1	1	1.5	2	2
Dry Beans/Peas	0.5	1	1	2.5	3	3
Starchy	1.5	2.5	2.5	2.5	3	3
Other	3.5	4.5	4.5	5.5	6.5	6.5

VEGETABLE SUBGROUPS (Cups per Week) (*continued*)						
Calorie Level	2,200	2,400	2,600	2,800	3,000	3,200
Dark Green	3	3	3	3	3	3
Orange	2	2	2.5	2.5	2.5	2.5
Dry Beans/Peas	3	3	3.5	3.5	3.5	3.5
Starchy	6	6	7	7	9	9
Other	7	7	8.5	8.5	10	10

Most vegetables are naturally low in fat and calories. None have cholesterol. Vegetables are important sources of many nutrients, including potassium, dietary fiber, folate, vitamin A, vitamin E, and vitamin C.

COUNT AS 1 CUP:

1 cup raw or cooked vegetables or vegetable juice
2 cups of raw leafy greens

Vegetables are organized into five subgroups, based on their nutrient content. Some commonly eaten vegetables in each subgroup are shown in the following table.

COMMONLY CONSUMED VEGETABLES

Dark Green	Orange	Dry beans/peas	Starchy	Other
Bok choy	Acorn squash	Black beans	Corn	Artichokes
Broccoli	Butternut squash	Black-eyed peas	Green peas	Asparagus
Collard greens	Carrots	Garbanzo beans (chickpeas)	Lima beans (green)	Bean sprouts
Dark green leafy lettuce	Hubbard squash	Kidney beans	Potatoes	Beets
Kale	Pumpkin	Lentils		Brussels sprouts
Mesclun	Sweet potatoes	Lima beans (mature)		Cabbage
Mustard greens		Navy beans		Cauliflower
Romaine lettuce		Pinto beans		Celery
Spinach		Soy beans		Cucumbers
Turnip greens		Split peas		Eggplant
Watercress		Tofu (bean curd made from soybeans)		Green beans
		White beans		Green or red peppers
				Iceberg (head) lettuce
				(continued)

COMMONLY CONSUMED VEGETABLES (*continued*)

Dark Green	Orange	Dry beans/peas	Starchy	Other
				Mushrooms
				Okra
				Onions
				Parsnips
				Tomatoes
				Tomato juice
				Vegetable juice
				Turnips
				Wax beans
				Zucchini

■ FRUIT GROUP: 1–2½ CUPS DAILY

The Fruit Group includes fruit or 100% fruit juice. The fruit may be fresh, canned, frozen, or dried; may be whole, cut-up, or pureed.

Most fruits are naturally low in fat, sodium, and calories. None have cholesterol. Fruits are important sources of many nutrients, including potassium, dietary fiber, vitamin C, and folate.

Only 100% fruit juices count as fruit servings. Most fruit drinks, punches, cocktails, and "ades" contain very little juice and a great deal of sugar. Beverages made from powdered fruit-flavored mixes or fruit-flavored carbonated beverages also do not count as fruit servings.

COUNT AS 1 CUP:
1 cup of fruit or 100 percent fruit juice
½ cup dried fruit

Fruits and vegetables contribute nearly half of the vitamin A and most of the vitamin C in Americans' diets. Because the vitamin A and C contents of fruits and vegetables vary greatly, menu planners must be especially careful to include sources of these nutrients in meals.

Vitamin A. Include one serving of an outstanding source at least every other day or at least one serving of a fair source each day. Outstanding sources of Vitamin A (at least 450 RAE per serving) include:
Organ meats (liver, giblets)
Yam, sweet potato
Braunschweiger
Frozen greens (collards, kale)

Pumpkin
Carrots
Spinach
Mixed vegetables, canned

Fair Sources of Vitamin A (at least 250 to 450 RAE per serving) include:
Instant cooked cereals, fortified
Various ready-to-eat cereals, fortified with vitamin A
Winter squash
Cantaloupe

For the vitamin A content of specific foods, see Appendix 7.

Vitamin C. Include one serving of an outstanding source or two servings of a fair source each day. Outstanding sources of Vitamin C (at least 45 milligrams per serving) include:
Peppers, green and red sweet pepper and hot chili
Kiwi fruit
Grapefruit juice
Orange or orange juice
Vitamin C-enriched fruit juices
Cantaloupe
Papaya
Strawberries
Brussels sprouts

Fair Sources of Vitamin C (at least 20 milligrams per serving) include:
Grapefruit
Kohlrabi
Raw pineapple
Broccoli
Tangerine/mandarin oranges
Mango
Tomato juice
Yam, sweet potato
Cauliflower
Frozen collard greens

▨ MEAT & BEANS GROUP: 2–7 OUNCE EQUIVALENTS DAILY

The Meat & Beans Group includes meat, poultry, fish, dry beans or peas, eggs, nuts, and seeds. Dry beans and peas are part of this group as well as the Vegetable Group.

Meat, poultry, fish, dry beans and peas, eggs, nuts, and seeds supply many nutrients. These nutrients include protein, B vitamins (niacin, thiamin, riboflavin, and B-6), vitamin E, iron, zinc, and magnesium.

COUNT AS 1 OUNCE EQUIVALENT:
1 ounce lean meat, poultry, or fish
1 egg
¼ cup cooked dry beans
1 tablespoon peanut butter
½ ounce of nuts or seeds
¼ cup tofu

Most meat and poultry choices should be lean or low-fat. If higher fat choices are made, such as regular ground beef (75% to 80% lean) or chicken with skin, the fat in the product counts as part of the discretionary calorie allowance. If solid fat is added in cooking, such as frying chicken in shortening or frying eggs in butter or stick margarine, this also counts as part of the discretionary calorie allowance. Select fish rich in omega-3 fatty acids, such as salmon, trout, and herring, more often. Fish, nuts, and seeds contain healthy oils, so choose these foods frequently instead of meat or poultry. The fat content of foods in this group varies greatly. The leanest cuts of meat include:

Beef roasts and steaks: round, loin, sirloin, chuck arm
Pork roasts and chops: tenderloin, center loin, ham
Veal: all cuts except ground
Lamb roasts and chops: leg, loin, fore shanks
Chicken and turkey: without skin
Fish and shellfish: most are low in fat; those marinated or canned in oil
  are higher in fat

■ **MILK GROUP: 2–3 CUPS DAILY**

The Milk Group includes fluid milk products and many foods made from milk. Foods made from milk that retain their calcium content—such as yogurt and cheese—are part of the group, while foods made from milk that have little to no calcium—such as cream cheese, cream, and butter—are not. Most milk group choices should be fat-free or low-fat.

Foods in the milk group provide calcium, potassium, vitamin D, and protein, which are vital for health and maintenance. Calcium is used for building bones and teeth and in maintaining bone mass. Milk products are the primary source of calcium in American diets. The intake of milk products is especially important to bone health during childhood and adolescence, when bone mass is being built. Diets rich in milk and milk products help build and maintain bone mass throughout the life-cycle. This may reduce the risk of osteoporosis.

Choose fat-free or low-fat milk, yogurt, and cheese. If milk or yogurt that is not fat-free or cheese that is not low-fat is chosen, the fat in the product counts as part of the discretionary calorie allowance. If sweetened milk products are chosen (flavored milk, yogurt, drinkable yogurt, desserts), the added sugars also count as part of the discretionary calorie allowance. For those who are lactose intolerant, lactose-free and lower-lactose products are available, such as hard cheeses and yogurt. Also, enzyme preparations can be added to milk to lower the lactose content. Calcium-fortified foods and beverages such as soy beverages or orange juice may provide calcium, but may not provide the other nutrients found in milk and milk products. For calcium equivalents, see Appendix 8.

COUNT AS 1 CUP:
1 cup milk
1 cup yogurt
1½ ounces natural cheese
2 ounces processed cheese

◼ OILS GROUP: 3–11 TEASPOONS DAILY

The Oils Group includes fats that are liquid at room temperature, like the vegetable oils used in cooking. Oils come from many different plants and from fish.

All fats and oils are a mixture of saturated fatty acids and unsaturated fatty acids. Solid fats contain more saturated fats and/or trans fats than oils. Oils contain more monounsaturated (MUFA) and polyunsaturated (PUFA) fats. Saturated fats, trans fats, and cholesterol tend to raise "bad" (low-density lipoprotein or LDL) cholesterol levels in the blood, which in turn increases the risk for heart disease. To lower risk for heart disease, cut back on foods containing saturated fats, trans fats, and cholesterol.

Most of the fats a person eats should be polyunsaturated (PUFA) or monounsaturated (MUFA) fats. Oils are the major source of MUFAs and PUFAs in the diet. PUFAs contain some fatty acids that are necessary for health, called "essential fatty acids."

The MUFAs and PUFAs found in fish, nuts, and vegetable oils do not raise LDL cholesterol levels in the blood. In addition to the essential fatty acids they contain, oils are the major source of vitamin E in typical American diets.

While consumption of some oil is needed for health, oils still contain calories. In fact, oils and solid fats both contain about 120 calories per tablespoon. Therefore, the amount of oil consumed needs to be limited to balance total calorie intake.

■ DISCRETIONARY CALORIES: 165–648 DAILY

A person needs a certain number of calories to keep the body functioning and provide energy for physical activities. Think of the calories you need for energy like money you have to spend. Each person has a total calorie "budget." This budget can be divided into "essentials" and "extras." Your discretionary calories are the "extras" that can be used on luxuries like solid fats, added sugars, and alcohol, or on more food from any food group.

Use discretionary calorie allowance to:

- Eat more foods from any food group than the food guide recommends.
- Eat higher calorie forms of foods-those that contain solid fats or added sugars. Examples are whole milk, cheese, sausage, biscuits, sweetened cereal, and sweetened yogurt.
- Add fats or sweeteners to foods. Examples are sauces, salad dressings, sugar, syrup, and butter.
- Eat or drink items that are mostly fats, caloric sweeteners, and/or alcohol, such as candy, soda, wine, and beer.

Tips for Menu Planning

Nutrition and selection tips for meal planning can be found in Appendix 11, "Exchange Lists for Meal Planning," listed under each food exchange list.

Study Guide Questions

A. List the *Dietary Guidelines for Healthy Americans 2005* focus areas:
1.
2.
3.
4.

     5.

     6.

     7.

     8.

     9.

B. Using MyPyramid and the Food Intake Patterns table, indicate how many servings from each group would be appropriate for a person requiring 1,800 calories per day:

Fruits

Vegetables

Grains

Meat & Beans

Milk

Oils

How many discretionary calories are allowed?

C. List at least three key nutrients found in each food group:

Grains

Vegetables

Fruits

Meat & Beans

Milk

D. An outstanding source of vitamin A should be included in the diet at least how often?

E. List at least three outstanding sources of vitamin A.

F. List at least two fair sources of vitamin A.

G. An outstanding source of vitamin C or two servings of a fair source of vitamin C should be included in the diet at least how often?

H. List at least three outstanding sources of vitamin C.

I. List at least two fair sources of vitamin C.

CHAPTER 2

ROUTINE DIETS

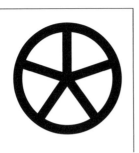

General Diet

Use

The General Diet is designed for people who require no dietary modifications and to reduce the risk of the development of chronic, nutrition-related diseases.

Adequacy

The suggested food plan includes food in amounts that will provide the quantities of nutrients recommended by the National Academy of Sciences for adults.

Diet Principles

1. The diet should provide adequate nourishment, variety, and color and be pleasing in texture and flavor.
2. The diet should incorporate the principles of the *Dietary Guidelines for Americans.*
3. The quantity of food selected from each food group should vary depending on the energy needs and preferences of the individual.

FOOD FOR THE DAY

Milk
2–3 cups — Milk may be fresh, dried, or evaporated; fat-free or reduced-fat; used as a beverage and in cooking; yogurt; cheese

Meat and Beans
2–3 servings
(total 2–7 ounce-equivalents) — Meat, poultry, fish, dry beans or peas, eggs, nuts, and seeds. Most meat and poultry choices should be lean or very lean

(continued)

FOOD FOR THE DAY *(continued)*

Fruits

1–2½ cups

Fruits may be fresh, frozen, canned, or dried; served whole, cut up, or pureed; 100% fruit juice

Vegetables

1–4 cups

Vegetables may be raw or cooked; fresh, frozen, canned, or dried/dehydrated; may be whole, cut-up, or mashed. Served plain or in mixed dishes; 100% vegetable juices

Choices of fruits and vegetables should include an outstanding source (or two fair sources) of vitamin C daily and an outstanding source of vitamin A at least every other day.

Grains

3–10 servings

Use whole-grain or enriched breads, whole-grain or enriched pasta, oatmeal, breakfast cereals, tortillas, grits, brown or wild rice, popcorn, cornbread, couscous, crackers, pretzels, buns, rolls. Eat at least 3 oz of whole-grain cereals, crackers, rice, or pasta every day

Oils/Fat

Use sparingly

Salad oils, margarine, butter, cream, mayonnaise, salad dressings, bacon. Make most of your fat sources from fish, nuts, and vegetable oils

Sweets/Desserts

1 or more servings

All sweets and desserts in limited amounts

Fluids

6–8 cups

Water and other fluids, such as coffee, tea, fruit or vegetable juice, lemonade, broth, or soup

---

SUGGESTED MENU PLAN FOR GENERAL DIET

(Select from foods described)

Breakfast

Fruit or juice

Whole-grain cereal with milk and/or egg

Whole-grain toast with margarine or butter

Hot beverage

Lunch or Supper

Soup or fruit or vegetable juice, if desired

Meat or meat substitute

Vegetable

Whole-grain bread with margarine or butter

Fruit or dessert

Milk

Dinner

Meat or meat substitute

Potato, pasta, or grain

Vegetable, cooked

Vegetable or fruit salad

Whole-grain bread with margarine or butter

Fruit or dessert

Milk

Nutritional Guidelines for Pregnancy and Lactation
(*Based on General Diet*)

Use

These nutrition guidelines provide increased amounts of protein, vitamins, and minerals needed by the pregnant or lactating woman.

Adequacy

The suggested food plan includes foods in amounts that will provide the quantities of all nutrients recommended by the National Academy of Sciences for the pregnant or lactating woman, depending on food choices. Special attention should be given to intakes of iron, folate, zinc, protein, and calcium to ensure adequacy. According to the *Dietary Guidelines for Americans 2005*, pregnant women should consume 600 μg/day of synthetic folic acid (from fortified foods or supplements) in addition to food forms of folate from a varied diet. It is not known whether the same level of protection could be achieved by using food that is naturally rich in folate.

Diet Principles

1. Weight gain during pregnancy should not be unduly restricted nor should weight reduction be attempted. The recommended weight gain during pregnancy for normal-weight women is 25–35 pounds. Underweight women are advised to gain 28–40 pounds, and overweight women 15–25 pounds. If excessive weight gain is a problem, the client's portion sizes and intake of "extra" foods will need to be evaluated.

2. The possible harmful effects of caffeine intake on a developing fetus are not yet fully understood. Pregnant and lactating women are advised to limit caffeine consumption to less than 300 mg per day. This would translate into less than 16 ounces of coffee per day.

3. Because of possible harmful effects on the developing fetus, it is advisable to avoid alcohol during pregnancy.

4. Women who are experiencing "morning sickness" or indigestion may find it helpful to eat "dry" meals, saving liquids for between meals; consume smaller, more frequent meals; eat high carbohydrate foods (toast, crackers, dry cereal); and avoid spicy foods or foods high in fat content. Individual tolerances vary, and women experiencing nausea should be encouraged to consume whatever foods and beverages they find appetizing.

5. For management of gestational diabetes, refer to "Gestational Diabetes Meal Plan" in Chapter 6.

FOOD FOR THE DAY

Food Group	Pregnancy	Lactation	Description
Milk	3–4 cups	3–4 cups	Milk may be fresh, dried, or evaporated; fat-free, low-fat, or reduced-fat; used as a beverage or in cooking; yogurt; cheese. The following each count as 1 cup (1 serving) of milk: 1 cup milk or yogurt, 1½ oz natural cheese such as Cheddar cheese or 2 oz processed cheese. Whole milk should be used only if additional calories are needed.
Meat and Beans	6–7 ounces	7–8 ounces	The following each count as 1 oz equivalent: 1 oz lean meat, poultry, or fish; 1 egg; ¼ cup cooked dry beans or tofu; 1 Tbsp peanut butter; ½ oz nuts or seeds.
Fruits	1½–2 cups	1½–2½ cups	Fruits may be fresh, frozen, or canned, served whole diced, or juice. Include at least 1 cup of vitamin-C rich fruit or vegetable daily.
Vegetables	2½–3 cups	2½–3½ cups	Vegetables may be fresh, frozen, or canned (including potatoes); served plain, in mixed dishes or as juice.
			2 cups leafy salad greens = 1 cup of vegetables.

A variety of vegetables are recommended with the following sub group recommendations for **cups per week.**

Dark green	3	3	Collard, turnip, and mustard greens, broccoli, spinach, romaine
Orange	2	2–2½	Carrots, sweet potatoes, winter squash and pumpkin
Legumes	3	3–3½	All cooked dry beans and peas and soybean products
Starchy	3–6	3–7	White potatoes, corn, and peas
Other	6½–7	6½–8½	All other vegetables

Grains	6–8 ounces	6–10 ounces	The following each count as 1 oz equivalent (1 serving) of grains: ½ cup cooked rice, pasta, or cooked cereal; 1 oz dry pasta or rice; 1 slice bread; 1 small muffin (1 oz); 1 cup ready-to-eat cereal flakes. At least half of the grain servings should be whole grain.
Oils/Fat	5–7 teaspoons	5–8 teaspoons	Oils and soft margarines without trans fats that are added to foods during processing, cooking or at the table.
Additional Foods	As needed for optimal weight gain of pregnancy	As needed to maintain milk supply and meet weight goals	Additional servings of the recommended foods or other foods may be served to meet individual energy needs.
Fluids	8–10 cups or more to satisfy thirst	10–12 cups or more to satisfy thirst	Fluoridated water and other fluids, such as fruit or vegetable juice, lemonade, broth, soup, decaffeinated coffee or tea.

For further reading, see Subcommittee on Nutritional Status and Weight Gain during Pregnancy, Subcommittee on Dietary Intake and Nutrient Supplements during Pregnancy, Committee on Nutritional Status during Pregnancy and Lactation, Food and Nutrition Board, Institute of Medicine, National Academy of Sciences. 1990. *Nutrition during Pregnancy*. Washington, D.C.: National Academy Press; and Work Group on Breastfeeding, American Academy of Pediatrics. 2005. Breastfeeding and Use of Human Milk. *Pediatrics* 115: 496–506.

Recommendations for Feeding Normal Infants

Use

These recommendations are designed for feeding infants, aged birth to 1 year, who require no special dietary modifications.

Adequacy

These recommendations will provide the quantities of nutrients recommended by the National Academy of Sciences for infants.

Diet Principles

Breastfeeding is considered the optimal infant feeding choice. Many families have misconceptions about breastfeeding and must be given accurate information in order to make an informed feeding choice. If families decide not to breastfeed their infant, iron-fortified formula is recommended.

■ ALL INFANTS

1. Feed infants when they give hunger cues rather than on a specific schedule. These cues include rooting, mouth opening, lip licking, placing hands to mouth, and motor activity. Breastfed infants nurse more often than formula-fed infants because breast milk is more quickly and easily digested than formula. (Infants may need to be awakened or prodded the first two to three days after birth due to drowsiness.)

2. Introduce solid foods when infants are developmentally ready using a spoon. This is usually between 4 and 6 months of age or when birth weight has doubled. Signs of developmental readiness include moving food from the front to the back of the mouth and swallowing it, sitting alone or with minimal support, reaching to grasp the spoon, and turning the head away to refuse food.

3. Fluoride supplements are not recommended for infants 6 months old or younger. From 6 months to 3 years, fluoride supplements are only needed if the amount of fluoride in drinking water is less than 0.3 parts per million.

■ BREAST-FED INFANT: BIRTH TO 6 MONTHS

1. During the early weeks of breastfeeding, mothers should be encouraged to have 8 to 12 feedings at the breast every 24 hours.

2. The American Academy of Pediatrics recommends that all breast-fed infants should receive 200 IU of oral vitamin D drops daily beginning during the first 2 months of life and continuing until the daily consumption of vitamin D-fortified formula or milk is 500 ml.

■ Bottle-Fed Infant: Birth to 6 Months

1. Iron-fortified formula is recommended and requires no vitamin or mineral supplementation if prepared with adequately fluoridated water.

2. Heating formula in the bottle in a microwave oven can cause mouth burns. Because the formula heats unevenly, the outside of the bottle can feel cool even though the contents are very hot.

■ AFTER AGE 4–6 MONTHS

1. Breast milk or iron-fortified formula is recommended for infants to age 1 year. Cow's milk in any form (whole, reduced-fat [2%],

low-fat [1%], or fat-free [skim]) and goat's milk should not be given to infants during their first 12 months.

2. A commercially prepared, single-grain infant cereal fortified with iron should be the first solid food introduced. The order of introduction of other solid foods is not important.

3. Introduce no more than one single-ingredient food at a time. Offer new foods at weekly intervals in order to identify food intolerances. The new food can be offered several days in a row.

4. Small, frequent feedings are preferable for infants. Let infants decide when they have had enough. "Full" cues include refusing to open mouth, turning head away, and spitting food out.

5. When infant foods are prepared at home, no salt or sugar should be added. Start with fresh or frozen foods as much as possible. Fruits canned in fruit juice and vegetables canned without salt can be used. The sugar and salt contents of many canned fruits and vegetables make them unsuitable for infants.

6. In the last several months of their first year, infants can progress from smooth foods to foods with more texture. Provide mashed foods first, followed by "chunky" foods. Offer cut-up soft table foods after infants have mastered eating chunky textures.

7. After the age of 12 months, foods should be the primary source of nourishment, even if a child continues to be breast- or bottle-fed.

8. By age 12 months, children make the transition from demand feeding to the family schedule of meals and snacks. By this time weaning from the bottle often occurs automatically as children become interested in eating table foods. Nursing from bottle or breast, if continued, should be in place of a scheduled snack and no longer given on demand. To protect children's teeth, frequent nursing from breast or bottle should not be permitted, and bottles should not be allowed in bed.

■ SAFETY CONCERNS

1. Honey should not be given to children under the age of 2 years. It may contain spores of the bacteria *Clostridium botulism*, which can produce a dangerous toxin in the gastrointestinal tracts of infants.

2. Water that has been in household pipes for more than 6 hours can contain lead. To ensure low levels of lead in formula and foods, prepare them with cold water that has run until it reaches its maximal coldness. Well water should be tested for nitrate and bacteria

levels. Boiling well water for formula is not recommended because nitrates and other substances can become concentrated.

3. Do not give infants round, slippery, and hard foods such as carrot slices, olives, hot dogs, peanuts, and hard candies. These foods can become lodged in the throat and block the air passage.

Nutrition Guidelines for Children

Use

These nutrition guidelines are designed for children aged 1–5 years who require no special dietary modifications.

Adequacy

The servings suggested for various age groups include foods in amounts that will provide the nutrients recommended by the National Academy of Sciences for the average child.

Diet Principles

1. The diet should provide adequate nourishment, variety, and color and be pleasing in texture and flavor.
2. Make mealtime enjoyable by serving a variety of textures and flavors in a pleasant setting. Children's appetites vary from day to day and go through phases of likes and dislikes. Serve small portions and allow children to ask for more food as they are ready. Avoid nagging, forcing, and bribing children to eat. Focusing attention on a child's poor appetite or eating problem will likely make the problem last longer.
3. Include snacks with high nutrient value in menu plans. The nutrient requirements of children cannot be met by meals alone because their small stomach capacity limits the amount of food they can eat at any one time.
4. Fat and cholesterol should not be limited in the diets of children under the age of 2 years; however, high fat foods with limited amounts of nutrients (pastries, gravies, fried foods, sweets) should be offered only in limited amounts.
5. The U.S. Dietary Guidelines recommend keeping total fat intake between 30–35% of calories for children 2 to 3 years of age and between 25–35% of calories for children and adolescents 4 to 18 years of age, with most fats coming from sources of

polyunsaturated and monounsaturated fatty acids, such as fish, nuts, and vegetable oils.

6. A sick child may regress in his or her level of performance, and this regression may progress throughout a long illness. For instance, a 6-year-old child may regress to the level of a 4- or 5-year-old so far as eating is concerned.

7. Excessive intake of milk tends to reduce the consumption of other foods. Lower fat milk is recommended for healthy children over the age of 2. Whole milk is recommended until 2 years of age.

8. For younger children it is important that meat be tender, moist, and cut into strips or bite-sized pieces. Young children like crisp finger foods; serve them regularly.

9. Highly seasoned foods may not be well accepted; use seasonings in moderate amounts.

10. Dieting at a young age can be dangerous to children's development, both physically and psychologically. If a child is overweight, maintaining weight during growth in height is recommended rather than encouraging weight loss unless a child is severely overweight. Any weight management efforts in children should occur under the monitoring of the family physician or a pediatric weight management program.

11. Vitamin and mineral supplements may be prescribed by a physician.

12. Children who routinely drink bottled waters may consume inadequate amounts of fluoride. Bottled water, which contains no fluoride, should not be offered as a frequent replacement for fluoridated tap water.

■ SAFETY CONCERNS

1. Toddlers and preschoolers can choke on medium to large pieces of food. Cut foods into small pieces and remove seeds, skin and small bones. Cut round foods like hot dogs, carrots and string cheese into short strips and chop whole grapes and berries into four pieces. Wait until closer to age 4 to serve risky foods like popcorn, pretzels, nuts, seeds, dried fruit and round or hard candy.

2. Peanut butter can stick in the mouth and be hard to swallow. Wait until children are closer to 2 years to offer peanut butter. Spread it thinly on crackers, bread or toast.

3. Require children to sit down when they eat to avoid choking and supervise them while eating.

FOOD FOR THE DAY

Milk

2 cups or equivalent for ages 2–8   Milk may be fresh, dried, or evaporated; fat-free, low fat,
3 cups for 9 years of age and older   or reduced fat; used as a beverage or in cooking;
                                             yogurt; cheese. The following each count as 1 cup
                                             (1 serving) of milk: 1 cup milk or yogurt, $1\frac{1}{2}$ ounces
                                             natural cheese such as Cheddar cheese or 2 ounces
                                             processed cheese. Whole milk should be used after age
                                             2 only if additional calories are needed.

Meat and Beans

2–4 ounces   The following each count as 1 ounce-equivalent: 1 oz lean
                                             meat, poultry, or fish; 1 egg; $\frac{1}{4}$ cup cooked dry beans or
                                             tofu; 1 Tbsp peanut butter; $\frac{1}{2}$ oz nuts or seeds.

Fruits

$\frac{3}{4}$–$1\frac{1}{2}$ cups   Fruits may be fresh, frozen, or canned, served whole,
                                             diced, or as juice[1]. Limit fruit juice to 4–6 ounces daily.
                                             Include at least $\frac{1}{2}$ cup vitamin-C rich fruit or vegetable
                                             daily.

Vegetables

$\frac{3}{4}$–$1\frac{1}{2}$ cups   Vegetables may be fresh, frozen, or canned (including
                                             potatoes); served plain, in mixed dishes or as juice.[1]
                                             1 cup leafy salad greens = $\frac{1}{2}$ cup of vegetables.

A variety of vegetables are recommended with the following sub group recommendations **per
week**.

Dark green (collard, turnip, and mustard greens, broccoli, spinach, romaine)	1 to $1\frac{1}{2}$ cups
Orange (carrots, sweet potatoes, winter squash and pumpkin)	$\frac{1}{2}$ to 1 cup
Legumes (all cooked dry beans and peas and soybean products)	$\frac{1}{2}$ to 1 cup
Starchy (white potatoes, corn, peas)	$1\frac{1}{2}$ to $2\frac{1}{2}$ cups
Other	$3\frac{1}{2}$ to $4\frac{1}{2}$ cups

Grains

3–5 ounce equivalents   The following each count as 1 oz-equivalent
                                             (1 serving) of grains: $\frac{1}{2}$ cup cooked rice, pasta, or cooked
                                             cereal; 1 oz dry pasta or rice; 1 slice bread; 1 small
                                             muffin (1 oz); 1 cup ready-to-eat cereal flakes. At least
                                             half of the grain servings should be whole grain.

Fats

3–4 teaspoons   Oils and soft margarines without trans fats that are added
                                             to foods during processing, cooking or at the table.

Fluids

$5\frac{1}{2}$–7 cups   Includes fluoridated water and other fluids, such as fruit or
                                             vegetable juice, lemonade, broth, or soup.

Additional foods

                                             Additional amounts of these foods or other foods may be
                                             served to meet individual energy needs.

[1] Juice should be full-strength to count as a serving.

SIZE OF SERVINGS FOR CHILDREN**

Food Group	1–2 years	3–5 years
Milk	½ cup	½–¾ cup
Fruits and Vegetables	¼–½ cup	½ cup
Grains		
Bread	½ slice	½ slice
Cornbread, biscuit, roll, or muffin	½ oz	½ oz
Cold dry cereal	¼ cup	⅓ cup
Hot cooked cereal	¼ cup	¼ cup
Pasta, noodles or other grains	¼ cup	¼ cup
Meat and Beans		
Meat, poultry, or fish	½–1 oz	½–1½ oz
Alternate protein product	1 oz	1½ oz
Egg	½ egg	½–¾ egg
Cooked dry beans	⅛–¼ cup	⅛–⅜ cup
Peanut butter	1–2 Tbsp	1–3 Tbsp
Nuts or seeds	½ oz	½–¾ oz

Based on USDA Child and Adult Care Food Program Meal Patterns. The smaller amounts are snack servings.
** This is the amount of food to have available. Individual children may eat smaller or larger servings to meet their energy needs.

Meeting Nutritional Needs of Older Adults

The aging process can affect the older adult in numerous ways: economic, functional, physiological and psychosocial. (24, 29, 32) These changes often influence not only nutritional status but also the risk for malnutrition. Dietetics professionals must be aware of the various physiological and clinically relevant changes that occur as people age. Studies show that food intake decreases even in the healthy older adult. (28, 42) Routine screening and assessment should be completed on a regular basis, as appropriate intake of food is important for successful, healthy aging. (9)

Russell and others have developed a Food Guide Pyramid for Older Adults at Tufts University. Potential nutritional problem areas identified for older adults are specifically addressed in this diagram. (30) Dietary adjustments to address the aging process must be considered.

Nutritional status is also affected when low income and food insecurity results in the older adult not having adequate means to obtain food. When a person's income is insufficient to meet basic needs, it is the responsibility of the dietetics professional to be proactive in helping the individual seek economic assistance. Awareness of the full range of options available (i.e., food stamps, home-delivered meals, congregate meals, food pantries) and the patterns of use within the community may ensure nutritional needs will be met. (31)

Many diseases or conditions that would be considered abnormal or alarming in younger adult populations are often seen as a part of the "normal aging process" in the older adult. (31) Use of nutrition care protocols can help with the identification of inadequate intake patterns and unintentional weight loss. (36) The dietetics professional must determine the underlying causes of weight changes (i.e., bowel elimination, uncontrolled disease processes, economic, oral, cognition, anorexia of aging, etc.)

Medications can affect intake, nutrient absorption, metabolism, and excretion, which can alter the nutritional status of an older adult. An assessment of all medications (prescribed, over-the-counter, and non-traditional) is important as food and drug interactions in the older adult remain largely under recognized. (10, 12)

Consider the following guidelines when prescribing and/or implementing food plans for older adults. Prior to prescribing a therapeutic diet, consider the person's quality of life, risk vs. benefits, and the impact the diet will have on the overall nutritional status of the older adult. This age group should be offered as liberal a diet as possible. (8)

1. Use the General Diet as much as possible, especially for people more than 70 years of age. People in long-term care facilities desire a homelike atmosphere where they feel loved and important. Serving popular, nutritious foods to some residents and not to others may cause anxiety, decreased food intake, and unhappiness.

2. If modifications are needed for the older person (especially the residents of long-term care facilities), the least restrictive diet is encouraged. Severely restricted diets and combination diets are not well accepted on a long-term basis, and are often the cause of malnutrition in the older adult.

3. Minor changes to a well-planned general diet may meet the needs of people with high blood cholesterol, diabetes, (8, 2) or for whom weight management is appropriate.

4. Research suggests that older adults with congestive heart failure can be controlled with drug therapy and a mild sodium restriction.

Low sodium diets may be poorly tolerated in this population leading to loss of appetite, hyponatremia, and/or confusion. (26)

5. A recent study by Grabowski et al. concluded that very obese
nursing home residents experience higher mortality early in their
stay, but this association diminishes over time with some evidence suggesting that a higher BMI may be protective among
long-stay residents. (16) Serving 1 percent milk, limiting cheese,
reducing portion size of desserts, and offering reduced sugar
sweeteners and condiments may be adequate for medical nutrition therapy.

6. Individualization is the key to dietary alterations for any person.
The menu plan should be personalized with a focus on physical,
mental, and social well-being. Choices from all the food groups
provide variety in the diet.

7. Food habits, influenced by ethnic, religious, and socioeconomic
factors, are important as older adults place much emphasis on
preserving their cultural traditions. Consider these factors when
planning meals and/or dietary modifications to maximize quality
of life.

8. Energy needs for the older adults are difficult to assess. (16) In
some cases, energy needs decrease as a result of decreased activity and lean body mass. In other cases, needs may increase due
to infection and stress. Meeting the needs of older adults is ex-
tremely challenging as requirements for many nutrients remain
the same or increase. (24) For this reason, foods need to be chosen carefully to ensure adequate nutrition. (41)

9. As part of the DRI, the RDA for protein needs of the older adult
is 0.8 g/kg of body weight/day. (44) However, some research has
indicated that protein needs may be as high as 1.0–1.25 g/kg of
high-quality protein/day. (27)

10. Dietary fat/lipid intake for older adults should be no more than
25–35% of total daily caloric intake. It is important to strike a
balance between palatability and adequate dietary intake to the
need for therapeutic fat restriction. Studies indicate that as age
increases, the importance of elevated serum cholesterol levels as
a risk for coronary heart disease decreases. (1, 33, 35) If there is
decreased tolerance to fats, avoid fried foods and decrease
amounts of fats added to or present in foods.

11. Intake of carbohydrates should compose 45–65% of total calories
for the older adult to protect protein from being used as an energy

source. Complex carbohydrates-whole grains, legumes, fresh fruits etc, should be a part of the older adult's daily intake. (24)

12. Intake of calcium and vitamin D should be emphasized in the older adult to aid in maintaining bone integrity. (17) For adults aged 51–70 years, the DRI for Vitamin D is 10 mcg and increases to 15 mcg for older adults. The recommended calcium intake for older adults—those over 50—is 1200 mg/day (22). Supplementation is sometimes needed. (24, 39)

13. Older adults may be less tolerant of milk and milk products, although small servings of milk (up to 8 oz per serving) may be tolerated. Milk products that have been fermented (i.e., buttermilk, cheese, or yogurt) or cooked (i.e., pudding, custard, cream soup, and sauces) are often tolerated. Lactase enzyme tablets may be used to aid digestion of fresh milk. The older adult should be encouraged to consume other calcium-rich food and beverage sources (dark green leafy vegetables, calcium-fortified foods/beverages) to help reduce the risk of osteoporosis. Restricting milk products may not be the answer if the older adult continues with such symptoms as diarrhea, abdominal cramping, etc. Consider medical causes such as gastroenteritis, *C. difficile*, colitis, and other conditions that may result in abnormal elimination patterns. Also consider possible effects of medications such as antibiotics, antacids, antidepressants, diuretics, laxatives, tranquilizers and those with large amounts of mannitol/ sorbitol.

14. Folate, (14) vitamin B-6 (24) and vitamin B-12 (15) intake and utilization may be affected in the older adult. Intake of these vitamins should be ensured either through fortified foods or supplements.

15. Encourage intake of iron-rich foods be taken in combination with vitamin C-rich foods. Do not take iron inhibitors-whether food or medication with meals. Avoid excessive or inappropriate iron supplementation due to potential side effects: gastrointestinal distress, iron overload, etc.

16. Liberal fluid intake promotes gastrointestinal function and prevents dehydration. A daily fluid intake of 30 ml/kg of body weight or a minimum of 1500 ml/day is often recommended for the older adult unless medical constraints prevent this amount. Numerous methods of calculations exist (24, 13, 40) therefore, select the method most appropriate. (31) A variety of beverages/foods may be used to meet fluid needs including broth, gelatin, ice cream, water, coffee, tea, carbonated beverages, and juices.

17. People who have difficulty chewing or swallowing may need adjustments in the consistency of the foods served to maintain adequate calories. (38) Meats may need to be chopped, ground, or pureed. Meats should be moist and well seasoned. Texture modifications should be individualized and used only when needed. For modifications, refer to the Consistency Altered Diets in Chapter 3.

18. Taste impairment is common in the older adult. Vegetables should be steamed, sautéed, or stir-fried to enhance their flavors. For those with dry mouth, offering very sweet or tart foods and beverages (lemonade or cranberry juice) may stimulate saliva production. Ice chips, sugar-free hard candy, gum or popsicles may also provide relief. Adding cream, gravy, sauces, soups, etc., to increase moisture of foods provided may help in the swallowing process. Numerous other artificial saliva preparations are available to help resolve/improve this problem.

19. Finger foods may be necessary for people with decreased dexterity. These foods are more easily consumed and increase independence. For more information, refer to the Finger Food Modification Diet in Chapter 11.

20. Food intake is improved when served at regular meal times, including a bedtime snack. Intake may be enhanced by serving the larger meal at midday and/or by serving smaller, more frequent meals. No more than 14 hours should elapse between a substantial evening meal and breakfast. Portion sizes at meals may vary based on an individual's nutritional needs.

21. Social contact in a pleasant environment may stimulate the appetite. This is important for people who live in long-term care facilities as well as people who live independently.

22. Evaluation for depression and alcohol use and their effects on the intake of the older adult must be assessed. Regular alcohol use may be associated with changes in absorption/utilization of vitamins B-6, B-12, and C; thiamin deficiency, decreased zinc absorption, and increased iron absorption. (25)

Study Guide Questions

A. Describe at least three ways in which aging can affect older adults.

B. List at least three options available to assist older adults in meeting their nutritional needs.

C. Describe in detail at least three guidelines for prescribing and/or implementing food plans for the older adult.

D. On one of your facility's diet spread sheets, plan a full one day General Diet menu for an older adult requiring 2,000 calories per day. Use MyPyramid and the Food Intake Patterns table as a guide. Include portion sizes.
    Note: This menu will be used later on as we review diet modifications.

E. During pregnancy, special attention should be paid to intakes of what five nutrients to ensure adequacy?

F. Describe in detail at least three diet principles to consider when developing menus for the average child.

G. What safety precautions should be taken when feeding a child?

CHAPTER 3

CONSISTENCY ALTERED
Diets

Altering the consistency of foods can greatly relieve eating problems related to chewing, managing food in the mouth, and swallowing. These problems may be due to stroke, head and/or neck injury, cancer, cerebral palsy, dementia, and other illness, or simply the result of aging. Aspiration (inhaling) of food into the lungs as a result of inadequate chewing and swallowing is now recognized as a major contribution to respiratory infections and pneumonia among institutionalized children and adults.

Difficulties in chewing and swallowing are often diagnosed as dysphagia, which occurs among all age groups but is seen more often among the elderly. It should be emphasized that the evaluation and treatment of dysphagia be done by a multidisciplinary team including a radiological physician, a swallowing therapist (speech language pathologist or occupational therapist), a dietitian, and a nurse.

Treatment of eating difficulties facilitates rehabilitation or maintenance of skills. Treatment may include oral motor exercises and changes in eating techniques, as well as altering the consistency of food and beverages. The dietitian and swallowing therapist will work closely together in assessing, recommending, and implementing the necessary texture changes on an individual client basis.

Before making major changes in food consistency or adding dietary supplements, all factors possibly contributing to eating problems should be evaluated. Food served must be well prepared, flavorful, and appealing. Appropriate assistive devices such as modified spoons, forks, and cups can make self-feeding easier. Proper positioning during eating and drinking is essential.

Principles of Consistency Alteration

1. The goals of consistency alteration are to allow clients to consume adequate nutrients and fluids and maintain nutritional status while reducing the risk of choking and aspiration. The chewing and swallowing ability should be evaluated before prescribing a consistency altered diet. The least restricted modification should be given.
2. Extensive individualization to meet energy, nutrient, and consistency of food and beverage needs is essential. Modifications in either solid foods or liquids or both may be necessary to achieve optimal nutritional status. Based on careful assessment of chewing and swallowing ability, diets can include combinations of unaltered solid foods, mechanically soft foods, and pureed foods. Clients vary greatly in chewing and swallowing ability.
3. The consistency of foods included in any modified diet can be altered. If no dietary modifications are needed for specific diseases, use the General Diet.
4. Monitor food and fluid intake closely as intake is often decreased. Foods of high nutrient density should be included when inadequate oral intake is observed. (See High Nutrient Diet in Chapter 11.)
5. Adequate fluid intake is essential. If clients will drink thickened beverages, they can be a source of fluids. Overly thickened beverages may be refused.
6. Fluid and nutritional supplementation may be necessary to ensure adequate hydration and nutritional status. Food intake should be evaluated and a comprehensive plan to increase food consumption should be in place before supplements are instituted.
7. Additional nutritional support or vitamin and mineral supplements may be needed for individuals with severe swallowing problems.
8. An individual's ability to chew and swallow may or may not improve. Periodic evaluation of chewing and swallowing capabilities should be conducted regularly with adjustments made in texture modification to meet the current skill level. Providing foods in a less modified texture allows the client to slowly progress to reach the highest level of independence. Reevaluation of swallowing abilities is beneficial to ensure clients are provided foods and beverages at the least restrictive level.

National Dysphagia Diets[1]

Level 1: Dysphagia Pureed Diet

Description

This diet consists of pureed, homogenous, and cohesive foods. Food should be "pudding-like." No coarse textures, raw fruits or vegetables, nuts, and so forth are allowed. Any foods that require bolus formation, controlled manipulation, or mastication are excluded.

Rationale

This diet is designed for people who have moderate to severe dysphagia, with poor oral phase abilities and reduced ability to protect their airway. Close or complete supervision and alternate feeding methods may be required.

Liquid Consistency (circle one)

Thin	Nectar-like	Honey-like	Spoon-thick

(Includes all unthickened
   beverages and supplements)

Food Textures for NDD Level 1: Dysphagia Pureed

Food Groups	Recommended	Avoid
Beverages	Any smooth, homogenous beverages without lumps, chunks, or pulp. Beverages may need to be thickened to appropriate consistency. **If thin liquids allowed, also may have:** Milk, juices, coffee, tea, sodas, carbonated beverages, alcoholic beverages, nutritional supplements. Ice chips.	Any beverages with lumps, chunks, seeds, pulp, etc.
Breads	Commercially or facility-prepared pureed bread mixes, *pregelled slurried* breads, pancakes, sweet rolls, Danish pastries, French toast, etc., that are gelled through entire thickness of product.	All other breads, rolls, crackers, biscuits, pancakes, waffles, French toast, muffins, etc.

(continued)

[1]The National Dysphagia Diets Level 1, Level 2, and Level 3 are (c)2003 American Dietetic Association. Used with permission.

(continued)

Food Groups	Recommended	Avoid
Cereals Cereals may have just enough milk to moisten.	Smooth, homogenous, cooked cereals such as farina-type cereals. Cereals should have a "pudding-like" consistency. **If thin liquids allowed, also may have:** Enough milk or cream with cereals to moisten; they should be blended well.	All dry cereals and any cooked cereals with lumps, seeds, chunks. Oatmeal.
Desserts	Smooth puddings, custards, yogurt, pureed desserts and soufflés. **If thin liquids allowed, also may have:** Frozen malts, yogurt, milk shakes, eggnog, nutritional supplements, ice cream, sherbet, plain regular or sugar-free gelatin.	Ices, gelatins, frozen juice bars, cookies, cakes, pies, pastry, coarse or textured puddings, bread and rice pudding, fruited yogurt. **These foods are considered thin liquids and should be avoided if thin liquids are restricted:** Frozen malts, milk shakes, frozen yogurt, eggnog, nutritional supplements, ice cream, sherbet, regular or sugar-free gelatin, or any foods that become thin liquid at either room (70°F) or body temperature (98°F).
Fats	Butter, margarine, strained gravy, sour cream, mayonnaise, cream cheese, whipped topping. Smooth sauces such as white sauce, cheese sauce or hollandaise sauce.	All fats with coarse or chunky additives.
Fruits	Pureed fruits or well-mashed fresh bananas. Fruit juices without pulp, seeds, or chunks (may need to be thickened to appropriate consistency if thin liquids are restricted). **If thin liquids allowed, also may have:** Unthickened fruit juices.	Whole fruits (fresh, frozen, canned, dried).
Meats and Meat Substitutes	Pureed meats. Braunschweiger. Soufflés that are smooth and homogenous. Softened tofu mixed with moisture. Hummus or other pureed legume spread.	Whole or ground meats, fish, or poultry. Nonpureed lentils or legumes. Cheese, cottage cheese. Peanut butter, unless pureed into foods correctly. Nonpureed fried, scrambled, or hard-cooked eggs.

Food Groups	Recommended	Avoid
Potatoes and Starches	Mashed potatoes or sauce, pureed potatoes with gravy, butter, margarine, or sour cream. Well-cooked pasta, noodles, bread dressing, or rice that have been pureed in a blender to smooth, homogenous consistency.	All other potatoes, rice, noodles. Plain mashed potatoes, cooked grains. Nonpureed bread dressing.
Soups	Soups that have been pureed in a blender or strained. May need to be thickened to appropriate viscosity. **If thin liquids allowed, also may have:** Broth and other thin, strained soups.	Soups that have chunks, lumps, etc.
Vegetables	Pureed vegetables without chunks, lumps, pulp, or seeds. Tomato paste or sauce without seeds. Tomato or vegetable juice (may need to be thickened to appropriate consistency if juice is thinner than prescribed liquid consistency). **If thin liquids allowed, also may have:** Thin tomato or vegetable juices.	All other vegetables that have not been pureed. Tomato sauce with seeds, thin tomato juice.
Miscellaneous	Sugar, artificial sweetener, salt, finely ground pepper, and spices. Ketchup, mustard, BBQ sauce and other smooth sauces. Honey, smooth jellies. Very soft, smooth candy such as truffles. **If thin liquids allowed, also may have:** Smooth chocolate candy with no nuts, sprinkles, etc.	Coarsely ground pepper and herbs. Chunky fruit preserves and seedy jams. Seeds, nuts, sticky foods. Chewy candies such as caramels or licorice.

Level 2: Dysphagia Mechanically Altered Characteristics

Description

This level consists of foods that are moist, soft-textured, and easily formed into a bolus. Meats are ground or minced into pieces no larger than one-quarter-inch; they are still moist, with some cohesion. All foods from NDD Level 1 are acceptable at this level.

Rationale

This diet is a transition from the pureed textures to more solid textures. Chewing ability is required. The textures on this level are appropriate for individuals with mild to moderate oral and/or pharyngeal dysphagia. Patients should be assessed for tolerance to mixed textures. It is expected that some mixed textures are tolerated on this diet.

Liquid Consistency (circle one)			
Thin	Nectar-like	Honey-like	Spoon-thick
(Includes all unthickened beverages and supplements)			

Food Textures for NDD Level 2: Dysphagia Mechanically Altered

(Includes all foods on NDD Level 1: Dysphagia Pureed in addition to the foods listed below)

Food Groups	Recommended	Avoid
Beverages	All beverages with minimal amounts of texture, pulp, etc. (Any texture should be suspended in the liquid and should not precipitate out.) (May need to be thickened, depending on liquid consistency recommended.) **If thin liquids allowed, also may have:** Milk, juices, coffee, tea, sodas, carbonated beverages, alcoholic beverages if allowed, nutritional supplements. Ice chips.	
Breads	Soft pancakes, well moistened with syrup or sauce. Pureed bread mixes, *pregelled* or *slurried* breads that are gelled through entire thickness.	All others
Cereals Cereals may have ¼ cup milk or just enough milk to moisten if thin liquids are restricted. The moisture should be well-blended into food.	Cooked cereals with little texture, including oatmeal. Slightly moistened dry cereals with little texture such as corn flakes, Rice Krispies, Wheaties, etc. Unprocessed wheat bran stirred into cereals for bulk. Note: if thin liquids are restricted, it is important that all of the liquid is absorbed into the cereal. **If thin liquids allowed, also may have:** Milk or cream for cereals.	Very coarse cooked cereals that may contain flax seed or other seeds or nuts. Whole-grain dry or coarse cereals. Cereals with nuts, seeds, dried fruit and/or coconut.
Desserts	Pudding, custard. Soft fruit pies with bottom crust only. Crisps and cobblers without seeds or nuts and with soft breading or crumb mixture. Canned fruit (excluding pineapple). Soft, moist cakes with icing or "slurried" cakes.	Dry, coarse cakes and cookies. Anything with nuts, seeds, coconut, pineapple, or dried fruit. Breakfast yogurt with nuts. Rice or bread pudding.

Food Groups	Recommended	Avoid
Desserts *(continued)*	Pregelled cookies or soft, moist cookies that have been "dunked" in milk, coffee, or other liquid. **If thin liquids allowed, also may have:** Ice cream, sherbet, malts, nutritional supplements, frozen yogurt, and other ices. Plain gelatin or gelatin with canned fruit, excluding pineapple.	**These foods are considered thin liquids and should be avoided if thin liquids are restricted:** Frozen malts, milk shakes, frozen yogurt, eggnog, nutritional supplements, ice cream, sherbet, regular or sugar-free gelatin, or any foods that become thin liquid at either room (70°F) or body temperature (98°F).
Fats	Butter, margarine, cream for cereal (depending on liquid consistency recommendations), gravy, cream sauces, mayonnaise, salad dressings, cream cheese, cream cheese spreads with soft additives, sour cream, sour cream dips with soft additives, whipped toppings. **If thin liquids allowed, also may have:** Cream for cereal.	All fats with coarse or chunky additives.
Fruits	Soft drained canned or cooked fruits without seeds or skin. Fresh soft/ripe banana. Fruit juices with small amount of pulp. If thin liquids are restricted, fruit juices should be thickened to appropriate viscosity. **If thin liquids allowed, also may have:** Thin fruit juices. Watermelon without seeds.	Fresh or frozen fruits. Cooked fruit with skin or seeds. Dried fruits. Fresh, canned, or cooked pineapple.
Meats, Meat Substitutes, Entrees Meat pieces should not exceed ¼ inch cube and should be tender.	Moistened ground or cooked meat, poultry, or fish. Moist ground or tender meat may be served with gravy or sauce. Casseroles without rice. Moist macaroni and cheese, well-cooked pasta with meat sauce, tuna-noodle casserole, soft, moist lasagna. Moist meatballs, meat loaf, or fish loaf. Protein salads such as tuna or egg without large chunks, celery, or onion. Cottage cheese, smooth quiche without large chunks. Poached, scrambled, or soft-cooked eggs (egg yolks should not be "runny" but should be moist and mashable with butter, margarine, or other moisture added to them).	Dry meats, tough meats (such as bacon, sausage, hot dogs, bratwurst). Dry casseroles or casseroles with rice or large chunks. Cheese slices and cubes. Peanut butter. Hard-cooked or crisp fried eggs. Sandwiches. Pizza.

(continued)

(continued)

Food Groups	Recommended	Avoid
Meats *(continued)*	(Cook eggs to 160°F or use pasteurized eggs for safety.) Soufflés may have small soft chunks. Tofu. Well-cooked, slightly mashed, moist legumes such as baked beans. All meats or protein substitutes should be served with sauces, or moistened to help maintain cohesiveness in the oral cavity.	
Potatoes and Starches	Well-cooked, moistened, boiled, baked, or mashed potatoes. Well-cooked shredded hash brown potatoes that are not crisp. (All potatoes need to be moist and in sauces.) Well-cooked noodles in sauce. Spaetzel or soft dumplings that have been moistened with butter or gravy.	Potato skins and chips. Fried or French-fried potatoes. Rice.
Soups	Soups with easy-to-chew or easy-to-swallow meats or vegetables: particle sizes in soups should be <½ inch. (Soups may need to be thickened to appropriate consistency, if soup is thinner than prescribed liquid consistency). **If thin liquids allowed, also may have:** All soups except those noted in **Avoid** column.	Soups with large chunks of meat and vegetables. Soups with rice, corn, peas.
Vegetables	All soft, well-cooked vegetables. Vegetables should be <½ inch. Should be easily mashed with a fork.	Cooked corn and peas. Broccoli, cabbage, Brussels sprouts, asparagus, or other fibrous, nontender or rubbery cooked vegetables.
Miscellaneous	Jams and preserves without seeds, jelly. Sauces, salsas, etc., that may have small tender chunks <½ inch. Soft, smooth chocolate bars that are easily chewed.	Seeds, nuts, coconut, sticky foods. Chewy candies such as caramel and licorice.

Level 3: Dysphagia Advanced Diet

Description

This level consists of food of nearly regular textures with the exception of very hard, sticky, or crunchy foods. Foods still need to be moist and should be in "bite-size" pieces at the oral phase of the swallow.

Rationale

This diet is a transition to a regular diet. Adequate dentition and mastication are required. The textures of this diet are appropriate for individuals with mild oral and/or pharyngeal phase dysphagia. Patients should be assessed for tolerance of mixed textures. It is expected that mixed textures are tolerated on this diet.

Liquid Consistency (circle one)

Thin	Nectar-like	Honey-like	Spoon-thick

(Includes all unthickened
   beverages and supplements)

Food Textures for NDD Level 3: Dysphagia Advanced

Food Groups	Recommended	Avoid
Beverages	Any beverages, depending on recommendations for liquid consistency. **If thin liquids allowed, also may have:** Milk, juices, coffee, tea, sodas, carbonated beverages, alcoholic beverages, nutritional supplements. Ice chips.	
Breads	Any well-moistened breads, biscuits, muffins, pancakes, waffles, etc. Need to add adequate syrup, jelly, margarine, butter, etc, to moisten well.	Dry bread, toast, crackers, etc. Tough, crusty breads such as French bread or baguettes.
Cereals Cereals may have ¼ cup milk or just enough milk to moisten if thin liquids are restricted.	All well-moistened cereals.	Coarse or dry cereals such as shredded wheat or All Bran
Desserts	All others except those on **Avoid** list. **If thin liquids allowed, also may have:** Malts, milk shakes, frozen yogurts, ice cream, and other frozen desserts. All others except those on **Avoid** list. **If thin liquids allowed, also may have:** Malts, milk shakes, frozen yogurts, ice cream, and other frozen desserts.	Dry cakes, cookies that are chewy or very dry. Anything with nuts, seeds, dry fruits, coconut, pineapple. Dry cakes, cookies that are chewy or very dry. Anything with nuts, seeds, dry fruits, coconut, pineapple.

(continued)

(continued)

Food Groups	Recommended	Avoid
Desserts *(continued)*	Nutritional supplements, gelatin, and any other desserts of thin liquid consistency when in the mouth.	**These are considered thin liquids and should be avoided if thin liquids are restricted:** Frozen malts, milk shakes, frozen yogurt, eggnog, nutritional supplements, ice cream, sherbet, regular or sugar-free gelatin or any foods that become thin liquid at either room (70°F) or body temperature (98°F).
Fats	All other fats except those on **Avoid** list.	All fats with coarse, difficult-to-chew, or chunky additives such as cream-cheese spread with nuts or pineapple.
Fruits	All canned and cooked fruits. Soft, peeled fresh fruits such as peaches, nectarines, kiwi, mangos, cantaloupe, honeydew, watermelon (without seeds). Soft berries with small seeds such as strawberries. **If thin liquids allowed, also may have:** Any fruit juices.	Difficult-to-chew fresh fruits such as apples or pears. Stringy, high-pulp fruits such as papaya, pineapple, or mango. Fresh fruits with difficult-to-chew peels such as grapes. Uncooked dried fruits such as prunes and apricots. Fruit leather, fruit roll-ups, fruit snacks, dried fruits.
Meats, Meat Substitutes, Entrees	Thin-sliced, tender, or ground meats and poultry. Well-moistened fish. Eggs prepared any way. Yogurt without nuts or coconut. Casseroles with small chunks or meat, ground meats, or tender meats.	Tough, dry meats and poultry. Dry fish or fish with bones. Chunky peanut butter. Yogurt with nuts or coconut.
Potatoes and Starches	All, including rice, wild rice, moist bread dressing, and tender, fried potatoes.	Tough, crisp-fried potatoes. Potato skins. Dry bread dressing.
Soups	All soups except those on the **Avoid** list. Strained corn or clam chowder. (May need to be thickened to appropriate consistency if soup is thinner than prescribed liquid consistency). **If thin liquids allowed, also may have:** All thin soups except those on the **Avoid** list. Broth and bouillon.	Soups with tough meats. Corn or clam chowders. Soups that have large chunks of meat or vegetables >1 inch.

Food Groups	Recommended	Avoid
Vegetables	All cooked, tender vegetables. Shredded lettuce.	All raw vegetables except shredded lettuce. Cooked corn. Nontender or rubbery cooked vegetables.
Miscellaneous	All seasonings and sweeteners. All sauces. Nonchewy candies without nuts, seeds, or coconut. Jams, jellies, honey, preserves.	Nuts, seeds, coconut. Chewy caramel or taffy-type candies. Candies with nuts, seeds, or coconut.

(NDD) Liquid Consistency Levels

Clients with swallowing difficulty can often handle thickened beverages better than normal thin fluids such as water, milk, or coffee. However, not everyone needs thickened liquids. Speech and occupational therapists use the following terms and measurement of thickness, or viscosity, to prescribe the appropriate consistency for liquids based on individual needs.

Definitions of Terms Used for Thickened Liquids

VISCOSITY BORDERS AND RANGES FOR THICKENED LIQUIDS	
Thin	1–50 cP
Nectar-like	51–350 cP
Honey-like	351–1,750 cP
Spoon-thick	>1,750 cP

*cP = Centipoise, the term for the measure of viscosity
Foods that are naturally nectar-like and do not require modification include: *Fruit nectars such as apricot and pear nectar, Tomato juice, and Buttermilk.*

© 2003, American Dietetic Association. Table used with permission.

Some manufacturers now put the viscosity measurement on their product labels. Avoid any liquid that changes thickness (viscosity) at room temperature (70°F) or body temperature (98°F). Examples include some nutritional supplements, milkshakes, eggnog, ice cream, and gelatin. A variety of commercial thickeners are available to modify liquids' consistencies. Follow the manufacturer's instructions to obtain the desired thickness.

SAMPLE MENU PLAN FOR NATIONAL DYSPHAGIA DIETS

(Select from foods for the day in the General Diet or any other diet. Follow the portion sizes for the appropriate diet using the textural modifications.)

Meal	General	Dysphagia Advanced	Dysphagia Mechanical	Dysphagia Pureed
Breakfast	Orange Juice*	Orange Juice*	Orange Juice*	Orange Juice, no pulp*
	Oatmeal or cornflakes*	Oatmeal or cornflakes*	Oatmeal or cornflakes*	Malt-O-Meal
	Fried Egg	Fried Egg	Scrambled Egg	Pureed Scrambled Egg
	Cinnamon Roll	Cinnamon Roll	Slurried Cinnamon Roll	Slurried Cinnamon Roll
	Margarine	Margarine	Margarine	Margarine
	Milk*	Milk*	Milk*	Milk*
Lunch or Supper	Baked Chicken	Ground Chicken	Ground Chicken, moistened	Pureed Chicken
	Baked Potato	Baked Potato-no skin	Baked Potato- no skin	Mashed Potatoes with butter
	Peas and Carrots	Peas and Carrots, tender	Pureed Peas and Carrots	Pureed Peas and Carrots
	Roll/Margarine	Roll/Margarine	Slurried Roll/Margarine	Slurried Roll/Margarine
	Apple Pie	Apple Pie	Apple Pie- no top crust	Pureed pie
	Milk*	Milk*	Milk*	Milk*
Dinner	Chicken Noodle Soup*	Chicken Noodle Soup*	Pureed Chicken Noodle Soup*	Pureed Chicken Noodle Soup*
	Crackers	Crackers in soup	Crackers pureed into soup	Crackers pureed into soup
	Grilled Cheese Sandwich	Grilled Cheese Sandwich	Pureed Grilled Cheese	Pureed Grilled Cheese
	Cherries	Cherries, canned	Pureed Cherries	Pureed Cherries
	Milk*	Milk*	Milk*	Milk*
Snack	Cookie	Cookie, soft	Soaked Cookie	Pureed Cookie

*If thin liquids restricted, thicken to appropriate consistency

Food and Beverage Preparation Tips

▓ THICKENERS FOR CONSISTENCY ALTERED FOODS

A variety of methods and special products are available to prepare a wide range of food consistencies. Thickeners for pureed foods and liquids include:

- For pureed foods:
    Commercial food thickeners, bread and cracker crumbs, instant potato flakes, instant infant cereal, flour, and instant pudding mixes are good nutritious thickeners. Commercial liquid thickening agents may also be useful.
- For liquids:
    Commercial thickeners, instant pudding mix, and instant potato flakes are good thickeners. Yogurt, applesauce, and puddings are also acceptable thickeners. Prethickened beverages are available.

Starch thickeners release approximately 100 percent of water during the digestion process. However, thickeners made from gums bind water even during digestion. Therefore, liquids thickened with gums do not help with hydration and might contribute to dehydration. Commercial food thickeners are made from starch and release most of the water during digestion. Client acceptance is always a concern. Introducing a new thickened beverage such as lemon-flavored thickened water or thickened fruit juice may be more acceptable than offering thickened coffee or milk, which would have a very different mouth feel than is usually expected with those flavors.

▓ PREPARATION OF TEXTURE ALTERED FOODS

Because diminished appetite is often present in individuals requiring texture modification, it is of utmost importance that the food be prepared to enhance its natural flavor. Every attempt should be made to make the food as palatable as possible. Minimize the total volume necessary to provide nutritional adequacy. Serve the food at the proper temperature. The foods should be served as separate entities and on attractive dishes with an appetizing presentation.

Use a food processor to achieve the desired consistency. Foods with a variety of consistencies can be prepared with the addition of very little liquid. The traditional blender usually requires more liquids, which dilutes nutrient density and increases the volume of foods.

Soaking or moistening recognizable foods in liquids, gravies, and slurries helps maintain their appeal. A slurry is a combination of a commercial thickener, common thickeners, or gelatin, with such liquids as milk, juice, or broth, and can be obtained by using 1–4 tablespoons of thickener or gelatin to 2 cups of liquid.

Cookies and cakes without nuts and chips can be soaked in milk. Bread or biscuits soaked in gravy or pancakes soaked in syrup or slurry are often well tolerated. A slurry can also be used to moisten and soften such foods as bread, cakes, cookies, or crackers. In addition, it is used to gel pureed foods. This allows an individual to consume food items that are not routinely part of the puree texture modification. Before serving a dry, crumbly food with added slurry, be sure the slurry soaks through the entire thickness of the food.

Method for Determining the Portion Sizes of Consistency Altered Foods

Foods often change in volume when they have been modified in consistency and texture. To ensure that nutritional adequacy is maintained, the following guidelines may be used when several portions of a consistency altered food are needed. Puree is used in this example.

1. Measure out desired number of servings into container for pureeing. Puree the food. Add any necessary thickener or liquid to obtain desired consistency. In most cases, it is desirable to maintain or increase the caloric value of consistency altered foods. When thinning foods use liquids that add to the nutritional value as well as the flavor of foods. Appropriate liquids include milk, fruit or vegetable juice, broth, gravy, cream sauce, and liquid nutrient supplements. Plain water is not recommended for thinning.
2. Measure the volume of the food after it has been pureed.
3. Divide the total volume of the pureed food by the original number of portions. This is the new portion size. Note: Some foods may have a smaller, rather than larger, portion after pureeing.
4. After dividing portions, foods must be reheated or chilled to serving temperature per HACCP guidelines.

Additional Resources

American Dietetic Association. 2000. *Manual of Clinical Dietetics,* 6th ed. Chicago: ADA.

American Dietetic Association. 2002. National Dysphagia Diet Task Force. *National Dysphagia Diet.* Chicago, IL: American Dietetic Association Press.

Department of Nutrition and Food Services, Alta. Bates-Herrick Rehabilitation Center and Hospital. 1990. *Dysphasia Dining*. Berkeley, CA, pp. 6, 25–29.

Felt, P. 1999. National Dysphagia Diet Project: The Science and the Practice. *Nutrition in Clinical Practice* 14 (Supplement): 60–63.

University of Iowa Hospitals and Clinics. 1995. *Recent Advances in Therapeutic Diets*, 5th ed. Ames: Iowa State University Press, pp. 23–26.

Study Guide Questions

A. Define *dysphagia*.

B. List at least three disciplines who should be involved in the evaluation and treatment of dysphagia.

C. Describe in detail four of the eight principles of consistency alteration.

D. List the four liquid consistencies.

E. Using your previously planned general menu for the older adult, show how this menu should be modified to accommodate persons on Dysphagia Advanced, Dysphagia Mechanical, and Dysphagia Pureed diets. Include portion sizes.

F. Describe the method for determining accuracy in portion sizes of consistency altered foods.

LIQUID DIETS
and Modifications

Clear Liquid Diet

Use

The Clear Liquid Diet is prescribed for preoperative or postoperative patients; for patients with an acute inflammatory condition of the gastrointestinal tract; in acute stages of many illnesses, especially those with fever; or in conditions when it is necessary to minimize fecal material (residue free).

Adequacy

This diet is inadequate in all nutrients. It should not be used more than 3 days without supplementation. Commercial clear liquid oral supplements may provide a source of protein and additional vitamins and minerals.

Note: A commercially prepared "defined formula diet" may be useful if a clear liquid regimen is necessary for more than 3 days or if the patient is seriously undernourished.

Diet Principles

This diet is composed of clear liquids. It is designed to provide fluids without stimulating extensive digestive processes, to relieve thirst, and to provide oral feedings that will promote a gradual return to a normal intake of food. Small servings may be offered every 2 or 3 hours and at mealtime. (Certain postoperative patients may be limited to tea and fat-free broth for one or more meals.)

FOOD FOR THE DAY

Fruits	Strained fruit juices: apple, cherry, cranapple, cranberry, crangrape, grape, orange, grapefruit
Soup	Fat-free clear broth and bouillon
Sweets/Desserts	Flavored and unflavored gelatin; popsicles; fruit ice made without milk; sugar, honey, syrup; hard candy; sugar substitutes
Fluids	Coffee, tea, carbonated beverages, approved for clear liquids such as Resource, Boost Breeze, Enlive, and NuBasics fruit beverage drinks

SUGGESTED MENU PLAN FOR CLEAR LIQUID DIET

(Select from foods described)

Breakfast

Fruit juice and/or broth
Gelatin
Tea or coffee

Lunch or Supper

Fruit juice
Broth
Gelatin
Tea or coffee

Dinner

Fruit juice
Broth
Gelatin
Tea or coffee

Between-Meal Nourishments

Fruit juice
Popsicle
Gelatin
Clear liquid nutritional supplement

Blenderized Liquid Diet

Use

The Blenderized Liquid Diet is prescribed for the postoperative patient, following the Clear Liquid Diet; for the acutely ill patient; and
for the patient who cannot chew or swallow solid or pureed food. It
may be prescribed to supplement a tube feeding.

Adequacy

Depending on the amount and choice of food eaten, this diet will tend to
be low in protein, calories, iron, thiamin, and niacin. It is recommended

for temporary use only. A multivitamin/mineral supplement should be ordered if a patient remains on the diet for more than 2–3 weeks.

Diet Principles

1. The Blenderized Liquid Diet includes foods that are liquid at body temperature and tolerated by the patient.
2. Because the diet typically includes many milk-containing foods, it may need modification for patients who do not tolerate lactose. Acidophilus milk or soy milk may be tolerated, or lactose-free nutrient supplement beverages can be useful.
3. If used over several weeks, low-fat dairy products should be included for patients with high blood cholesterol levels. Modifications in carbohydrate levels may also be necessary for people with diabetes mellitus or hypoglycemia.

FOOD FOR THE DAY

Milk	As a beverage and in cooking; milk in milk drinks, such as eggnog, milk shake, or malted milk; in strained cream soups; yogurt without fruit pieces or seeds

Note: Do not serve raw egg. Use blended baked custard, soft custard with added milk, or a commercial mixture that is pasteurized.

Meat and Beans 2–3 servings (total 2–7 ounces)	Eggs in eggnog, soft custard; pureed meat added to broth or cream soup
Fruits 1 cup or more	Citrus and other fruit juices; pureed fruit without seeds
Vegetables 1 cup or more (including potatoes)	Potato, strained in cream soups; other mild-flavored vegetables, such as asparagus, carrots, green beans, peas, or spinach, strained and combined with clear broth, cream soup, plain or flavored gelatin; vegetable juices

Choices of fruits and vegetables should include one outstanding source of vitamin C (or two fair sources) daily and one outstanding source of vitamin A at least every other day.

Grains 1 or more servings	Refined or strained cooked cereals that have been thinned with hot milk or hot half-and-half
Oils/Fat 4 servings	Vegetable oils, fortified margarine or butter, cream, or non-dairy creamer
Sweets/Desserts	Sugar, honey, sugar substitutes, syrup
Fluids	Coffee, tea, carbonated beverages
Other	Broth or strained cream soup combined with allowed strained vegetables; soft or baked custard, flavored and unflavored gelatin, plain ice cream, pudding, sherbet, popsicles, flavorings and mild spices in moderation; nutritional supplements

---

SUGGESTED MENU PLAN FOR BLENDERIZED LIQUID DIET

(Select from foods described)

Breakfast

Fruit juice
Thinned, cooked cereal with cream, sugar
Milk or milk beverage

Lunch or Supper

Soup *
Pureed fruit
Fruit juice
Dessert
Milk or milk beverage

Dinner

Soup*
Pureed fruit
Yogurt
Milk or milk beverage

Between-Meal Nourishments

Milk or milk beverage
Fruit juice
Pureed fruit
Yogurt
Nutritional supplement

---

*Soups may be fortified with dry milk, pureed meat and vegetables, and a fat serving.

Post-Surgical Diet

Use

The Post-surgical Diet is prescribed when it is decided the post-surgical patient is ready to have some whole foods but is not yet ready for a routine diet.

Adequacy

Depending on the amount and choice of food eaten, this diet will tend to be low in protein, calories, iron, thiamin, and niacin. It is recommended for temporary use only.

Diet Principles

In addition to foods allowed on the Blenderized Liquid Diet the patient may have soft-cooked, or scrambled eggs; cottage cheese; baked (no skin), boiled, mashed, or creamed potatoes; refined cooked cereals; quick-type oatmeal; toasted white bread; soda crackers. Other foods from a routine diet may be added as the patient is able to tolerate them.

Enteral Feeding

Use

Enteral feeding may be prescribed for patients who are physically or psychologically unable to take food by mouth in amounts that will support adequate nutrition. Some enteral feeding products are palatable enough to be used as oral supplements to supply additional calories and/or other nutrients to patients who are able to consume some, but not enough, food by mouth. Enteral feedings should be administered under the close supervision of a physician and monitored by a dietitian.

Adequacy

Many enteral feedings will be nutritionally adequate when given in recommended amounts, but it is important to evaluate each patient individually.

Diet Principles

1. **Selection**. Choice of an enteral feeding product depends on the medical and nutritional needs of the patient as determined by the physician and dietitian. In addition to the many lactose-free standard formulas, there are those specifically designed for digestive and absorptive disorders, stress, trauma, and renal or hepatic disease. Availability of a specific formula will vary among institutions.
2. **Administration**. Access to the stomach or small intestine is gained via a very small diameter, flexible feeding tube. The tube may be placed nasogastrically, nasojejunally, or via esophagostomy, gastrostomy, or jejunostomy. Formula is delivered through the tube by gravity flow or by use of a metered pump. The concentration, rate, and volume of formula given depend on individual factors, such as nutritional status, body size, and type of formula. The feeding is initiated at a slow rate and/or a reduced concentration and then gradually advanced as tolerated to the predetermined rate and strength necessary to meet nutritional needs. A multivitamin/mineral supplement is needed if the volume of formula does not meet the recommendations of the Food and Nutrition Board, National Academy of Sciences.
3. **Complications**. The major complications of enteral feeding are due to too concentrated a formula or too rapid a rate of advancement, poor positioning of the patient, and in some cases, bacterial contamination by improper handling and feeding practices. Results can include diarrhea, constipation, aspiration, electrolyte imbalance, dehydration, hyperglycemia, and azotemia. Frequent

monitoring of hydration status, residual volume in stomach, blood and urine chemistries, and physical signs is important to avoid complications. Meticulous care in selecting, mixing, handling, storing, and administering feedings is essential.

4. **Information** about specific enteral feeding formulas can be obtained from company representatives.

Study Guide Questions

A. List three reasons why the Clear Liquid Diet may be prescribed.
B. List at least eight specific items that can be included on the Clear Liquid Diet.
C. Plan a full one-day menu for an individual on a Blenderized Liquid Diet.
D. List at least four foods that may be added to the Blenderized Liquid Diet as post-surgical clients are able to tolerate them.
E. List four factors that should be considered when using enteral formulas.

CHAPTER **5** _____

DIETS FOR
_____
Weight Management

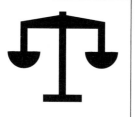

There are a record number of adults and children with weight management concerns in America today. The results from the 1999–2000 National Health and Nutrition Examination Survey (NHANES) revealed that nearly 66% of adults in the United States are overweight and 30.5% are considered obese. The economic impact has been estimated at near $117 billion when all health aspects are taken into consideration. This is comparable to the economics of cigarette smoking in the United States.

Being overweight or obese are known risk factors for type 2 diabetes, cardiopulmonary disease, stroke, hypertension (high blood pressure), gallbladder disease, osteoarthritis, sleep apnea, and some forms of cancer. Obesity is also associated with hyperlipidemia (high blood cholesterol), complications associated with pregnancy, irregular menses, hirsutism (excess body and facial hair), stress incontinence, depression, and increased surgical risk if such procedures are needed. Given the above, obesity is the second preventable cause of death in the United States.

Being overweight or obese are described as having an excess of body weight according to standards for height. A more specific measurement would be using Body Mass Index (BMI) (see Appendix 5). A BMI of 25 to 29.9 kg/m^2 is considered overweight. Obesity is defined as a BMI of $\geq$ 30 kg/m^2 (see Appendix 6 for diagnostic terms). In the last decade, these groups have risen 54.9% between men and women in their 20's. In older adults, higher BMI is associated with lower mortality rates. (23)

Treatment for being overweight or obese includes diet and behavior therapy. Exercise is a key part of the treatment and should be customized to the client's ability. Client motivation should also be evaluated as well as the individual's understanding of the causes of obesity

55

and how obesity contributes to disease. The overall strategy for treatment of overweight/obesity is outlined in figure 5.1.

Weight Management Diet

Use

The use of calorie-controlled diets for weight management follow the principals of the General Diet, except that the portion sizes and fat content are decreased based on the client's nutritional needs and weight management goals. The diet content is similar to the Cholesterol/Saturated Fat Restricted Diet outlined in Chapter 7. Keep in mind that diet alone will not produce achievable sustainable results. Weight management includes diet therapy, physical activity, and behavior therapy. Pharmacotherapy is used after all other avenues have been tried for at least 6 months. The use of this diet can do the following:

- Promote weight loss by reducing calorie needs by 500–1,000 calories per day
- Promote weight maintenance by providing adequate calories based on expenditure once a weight loss goal is met
- Achieve optimal serum lipid levels (cholesterol, HDL and LDL cholesterol, and triglycerides)
- Prevent long-term complications such as hypertension (high blood pressure), cardiovascular disease, diabetes
- Improve overall health through optimal nutrition

Adequacy

Very low calorie diets do not meet energy requirements or nutrient requirements and should only be used under supervision. Calorie levels less than 1,200 for women and 1,500 for men should be discouraged. These levels lack adequate intake to meet vitamin and mineral needs. A multivitamin/mineral supplement should be considered. Diets that promote weight loss are based on the General Diet with a reduction of 500–1,000 calories per day. The diet should be based on the individual's nutritional needs and anticipated energy output.

Diet Principals

1. Maintain a healthy weight either by weight loss or weight maintenance. A 10% loss of current body weight is a goal to promote a lower blood sugar, blood cholesterol, and blood pressure.

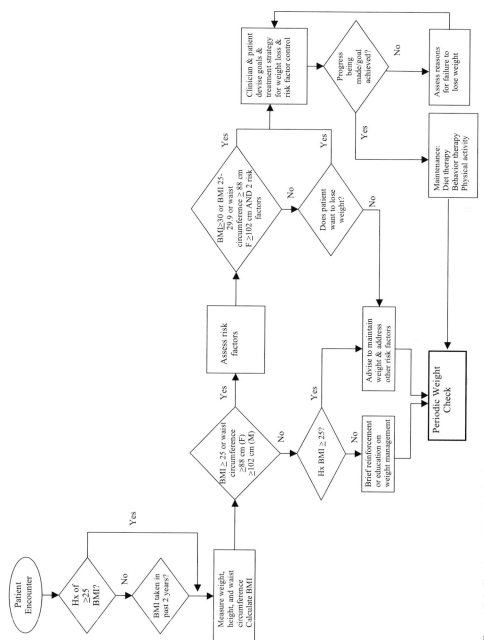

Figure 5.1. Treatment Algorithm for Assessment of Overweight and Obesity. (Source: National Heart, Lung, and Blood Institute [part of the National Institutes of Health and U.S. Dept. of Health and Human Services] and North American Association for the Study of Obesity. Oct 2000. *The Practical Guide: Identification, Evaluation, and Treatment of Overweight and Obesity in Adults.*)

2. Prevent additional weight gain which is critical for health goals.
3. Establish a pattern of safe weight loss equaling 1–2 pounds per week. When rapid weight loss occurs, the chance of regain is greater.
4. Support lifestyle, behavior modification, exercise and diet changes which are an ongoing process that last indefinitely.
5. Monitor food intake and weight by way of food diary or other means of recording.
6. Exercise a minimum of 30 minutes at least 5 days a week to help promote weight loss or weight maintenance.
7. Choose heart healthy foods that are moderate to small in portion size to meet weight loss goals.
8. Spread meals and snacks throughout the day to prevent hunger periods.
9. Include protein and small amount of healthy fat with meals to increase satiety and decrease between-meal hunger.
10. Drink at least 64 ounces of calorie-free liquids per day to help maintain hydration as well as to promote a sense of fullness to aid with weight loss.

Weight loss with the elderly population should be evaluated based on benefit for long term outcomes. Weight loss with children should be monitored by a health care team.

SUGGESTED MENU PLAN FOR WEIGHT MANAGEMENT

 Refer to the suggested menu plan for the Cholesterol/Saturated Fat Restricted Diet in chapter 7.

Calorie-Controlled Diets

A diet prescription may include a calorie range, such as 1,200–1,500 calories per day. Use the number of exchanges listed under each calorie pattern as the least and most exchanges to include from each exchange list to keep energy intake within the recommended range. Use Appendix 11, "Exchange Lists for Meal Planning," for reference in meal planning.

CALORIE LEVEL	1,000	1,200	1,600	1,800	2,000	2,200	2,800	2,000–2,200[a]
Total Food Exchanges								
Grains	3	4	5	6	6	7	10	6–7
Meat and Beans	2	3	5	5	5.5	6	7	6
Vegetable	2	3	4	5	5	6	7	5
Fruit	2	2	3	3	4	4	5	4
Milk, fat-free	2	2	3	3	3	3	3	4
Oils/Fat	3	4	5	5	6	6	8	6
Discretionary Calories	165	171	132	195	267	290	410	267
Sample Meal Pattern								
Breakfast								
Grains	1	2	2	2	2	2	3	2
Meat and Beans	0	0	1	1	1	1	1	1
Fruit	1	1	1	1	1	1	1	1
Milk, fat-free	½	½	1	1	1	1	1	1
Oils/Fat	1	1	1	1	2	2	2	2
Lunch or Supper								
Grains	1	1	1	2	2	2	3	2
Meat and Beans	1	1	2	2	2	2	3	2
Vegetable	1	2	2	2	2	2	3	2
Fruit	0	0	1	1	1	1	1	1
Milk, fat-free	1	1	1	1	1	1	1	1
Oils/Fat	1	1	2	2	2	2	3	2
Dinner								
Grains	1	1	2	2	2	2	3	2
Meat and Beans	1	2	2	2	2.5	3	3	3
Vegetable	1	1	1	2	2	2	2	2
Fruit	1	1	1	1	1	1	2	1
Milk, fat-free	0	0	0	1	1	1	1	1
Oils/Fat	1	2	2	2	2	2	3	2
Snack								
Grains	0	0	0	0	0	1	1	0–1
Vegetable	0	0	1	1	1	2	2	1
Fruit	0	0	0	0	1	1	1	1
Milk, fat-free	½	½	1	0	0	0	0	1
Discretionary Calories[b]	165	171	132	195	267	290	410	267

[a]2,000–2,200 calorie diet that includes 4 cups milk is included for an adolescent or during pregnancy.

[b]Discretionary Calorie Allowance is the remaining amount of calories in a food intake pattern after accounting for the calories needed for all food groups using forms of foods that are lean, fat-free or low-fat and with no added sugars.

[c]Information derived from USDA MyPyramid, refer to chapter 1.

Additional Resources/Websites

American Council for Fitness & Nutrition: www.acfn.org
American Dietetic Association: www.eatright.org
American Medical Association: www.ama-assn.org
American Obesity Association: www.obesity.org
National Center for Health Statistics: www.cdc.gov/nchs
National Health Information Center: www.health.gov/NHIC
North American Association for the Study of Obesity: www.naaso.org
President's Council on Physical Fitness and Sports: www.fitness.gov
Shape up America: www.shapeupamerica.org
Weight-control Information Network, US Department of Health and
    Human Services: http://win.niddk.nih.gov

Bariatric/Gastric Bypass Diet

Use

The Bariatric/Gastric Bypass diet is for obese clients who have undergone weight loss surgery. The Roux-en-Y is the most common bariatric surgery and produces weight loss with a combination of malabsorption and restriction principles. It is imperative to determine what type of bariatric surgery was performed as the diet and nutrition plan could vary; the diet described here is specifically for the Roux-en-Y procedure.

Adequacy

This diet is not adequate in any nutrient without proper supplementation. Clients are at significant risk of malnutrition because the amount of food consumed is severely limited, and less small intestinal area is available for absorption of nutrients. High protein supplements may be required for 4–6 months. Life-long supplements are commonly prescribed for multivitamin/ minerals, calcium, iron and sublingual vitamin B-12.

Diet Principles

1. Eat 1–3 "meals" per day, snack rules vary.
2. Consume a maximum of 2–4 Tbsp per "meal."
3. Consume a minimum of 60 grams of protein per day.
4. No liquids with meals and 30 minutes before and after eating solids.
5. Take small bites, chew 25–30 times per bite.
6. Consume at least 64 ounces of water per day.
7. Do not use straws.

DIET PROGRESSION FOLLOWING ROUX-EN-Y PROCEDURE

Days 1–10	Clear liquids only (water, broth, sugar-free gelatin). Ensure UGI is cleared (no leaks) before progressing.
Days 11–31	Add powder and/or liquid protein supplements to provide 50–60 g protein/day. If mixed with milk, count as a "meal." Gradually add soft, moist proteins; texture level (ground, pureed) varies by program and individual tolerance, i.e., eggs, cottage cheese, refried beans, milk, yogurt, string cheese, bean soups, poultry, tofu May add **small** amounts of fats to provide moisture.
Months 2–4	Eat **protein first**; as satiety allows, add fruits (peeled, non-citrus) and cooked vegetables (non-starchy), as well as hard cheeses and peanut butter.
Month 5	Eat **protein first**; as satiety allows, add fruits and/or vegetables second, then add carbohydrates if room. Overcook pasta and rice to prevent swelling. (The time period for adding carbohydrates varies by program.) May attempt red meats (beef, pork, lamb), digestion is difficult and may not be tolerated even 12 months out.
Month 6 and Beyond	Continue small portions; may eventually be able to tolerate 1–1½ cups/meal. Work up to 1,000 calories and include foods from all food groups. Continue goal of 60 g protein and 64 oz water. Pay close attention to feelings of hunger and satiety. Do not eat due to psychological hunger (angry, lonely, tired, stress, boredom, etc.). Make physical activity a priority.
Supplement Suggestions	For protein powders, a whey protein isolate is preferred; lactose-free is also desirable. Immediately post-op: Multivitamin/minerals and calcium: sugar-free and chewable for the first 6 weeks, then tablets are acceptable. Begin at 6 weeks post-op: ferrous fumerate and Vitamin B-12 (must be sublingual, nasal, or intramuscular).
Nutrition Facts Label Goals (All Stages)	Be sure to adjust serving sizes to amounts consumed. 2 g sugar/serving and 15 g sugar/meal. Note: Sugar substitutes, and natural lactose and fructose are generally well tolerated. 25 g total carbohydrate/serving 20 g fat/day

Additional Resources

Foster G., Nonas C. 2004. *Managing Obesity: A Clinical Guide.* Chicago, IL: American Dietetic Association.

Greiman L. 2005. Considerations and questions to ask when you don't routinely work with bariatric surgery patients. *ADA's Weight Management DPG Newsletter.* Spring; 2(4).

Marcason W. 2004. What are the dietary guidelines following bariatric surgery? *J Am Diet Assoc.* 104(3):487–488.

Websites

American Society for Bariatric Surgery: www.asbs.org
Bari MD: www.barimd.com
Obesity Help, Inc.: www.obesityhelp.com
Remedy MD: www.remedymd.com
Weight Control Information Network: win.niddk.nih.gov/publications/labs.htm

Study Guide Questions

A. 1. What percentage of adults in the United States are considered overweight?
    2. What percentage of adults in the United States are considered obese?
    3. What are the costs (in billions of dollars) associated with adults being overweight and obese?
B. List at least six health-related problems associated with being overweight or obese.
C. Weight management includes what three factors?
D. Using the exchanges listed in the Calorie Controlled Diet, plan a full one-day menu for a client on a 1,200-calorie diet.
E. Using the exchanges listed in the Calorie Controlled Diet, plan a full one-day menu for a client on a 1,800-calorie diet.

CHAPTER 6 _____

Diets for
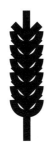
Diabetes

There are approximately 18 million Americans with diabetes mellitus. Of this population, 90–95% has type 2 diabetes and the remaining 5–10% has type 1 diabetes. Diabetes is a disease in which the body does not produce or properly use insulin. Insulin is a hormone that is needed to convert sugar, starches, and other foods into energy needed for daily life. If the carbohydrate is unable to be transported into the cell, the carbohydrate remains in the blood stream and produces a state of hyperglycemia (high blood sugar). This prolonged state causes damage to the body by macrovascular (large vessel) and microvascular (small vessel) damage.

Type 1 diabetes (previously known as *juvenile diabetes* or *insulin dependent diabetes* or *IDDM*) is an auto-immune disease that affects the pancreas in a way that it does not release insulin. Insulin is required for a type 1 diabetic to survive; injections are given to replace the insulin. Currently there is no known cure for type 1 diabetes, although research is consistently underway.

Type 2 diabetes (previously known as *adult onset diabetes* or *non-insulin dependent diabetes* or *NIDDM*) is a disease that progressively results in the inability of the pancreas to function properly. Over time, the pancreas production of insulin diminishes. Type 2 diabetes may require medication to control blood sugar. This may include oral medication and/or insulin. Once a type 2 diabetic starts an insulin program, the person does not become a type 1 diabetic; the description for this patient is "Type 2 diabetic requiring insulin."

There is also a new population that is not considered diabetic but has blood sugars that are higher than normal. This group is termed *pre-diabetic*. There are 41 million people with pre-diabetes in addition to the 18 million noted above. Usually diet, exercise, and weight management can prevent or delay the onset of type 2 diabetes.

Another type of diabetes is called *gestational diabetes*. This type of diabetes only occurs during pregnancy. After delivery of the baby, the blood sugar returns to normal. Women who have gestational diabetes are at a higher risk for type 2 diabetes. Meal planning, exercise, and possibly medication are used to control the blood sugar during pregnancy.

Consistent Carbohydrate Diet

Use

The Consistent Carbohydrate Diet is an outline for meal planning for the client with diabetes mellitus. This diet follows the principles of the General Diet but provides consistent carbohydrate intake at meals. The goals of nutrition therapy in treating diabetes are:

- Maintain as near normal blood glucose levels as possible
- Achieve optimal serum lipid levels (cholesterol, HDL and LDL cholesterol, and triglycerides)
- Provide adequate energy to achieve and maintain a reasonable body weight in adults and to support growth during pregnancy and childhood
- Prevent and treat short-term complications such as hyper- or hypoglycemia (high or low blood sugar) and long-term complications such as renal (kidney) disease, cardiovascular disease, neuropathies (nerve damage), and amputation
- Improve overall health through optimal nutrition

Adequacy

The suggested food plan includes foods in amounts that will provide the quantities of nutrients recommended by the National Academy of Sciences for adults. Meal plans with less than 1,200 calories may be low in vitamins and minerals and are generally not recommended. The need for nutrient supplementation should be evaluated.

Diet Principles

The following principles are based on the Clinical Practice Recommendations from the American Diabetes Association *Diabetes Care 2006 Volume 29* (Supplement 1):

1. **Individualization**. Individualization of treatment for patients with diabetes is essential. The effect of medical nutrition therapy

on blood glucose and serum lipid levels (especially triglycerides and LDL cholesterol) must be evaluated and modified, if necessary. The dietary program and self-management plan must take into consideration the ability and willingness of the client with diabetes to follow through with recommendations. The plan should be sensitive to cultural, ethnic, and financial considerations. Reinforcement of teaching and encouragement are usually necessary over an extended period of time.

2. **Energy**. The caloric value of meal plans must provide adequate energy to achieve and maintain a desirable or reasonable weight. Weight reduction of 10–20 pounds can improve blood glucose levels as well as blood pressure in most obese people with type 2 diabetes. For individuals with diabetes that are within a desirable weight range, caloric intake must match expenditure to maintain normal weight. For the person below desirable weight, caloric intake must allow for appropriate weight gain.

3. **Carbohydrate.** Carbohydrates affect the blood sugar 100 percent of the time whether you have diabetes or not. Nutritional recommendations advocate 50–60% of total calories from carbohydrates. Carbohydrates include four main groups of food: (1) starches, (2) fruit and fruit juices, (3) milk and milk products, and (4) sweets, desserts, and other carbohydrates. These foods affect the blood sugar in the same manner. The pancreas releases insulin based on the amount of carbohydrate that is consumed. For those who require medication, the right dose is given based on the assessment of the individual. The total amount of carbohydrate consumed is more important than the source of the carbohydrate. Research shows that sugars such as sucrose (table sugar), fructose, corn syrup, and honey have no more effect on blood glucose levels than other carbohydrates. Monitoring blood glucose after meals can help evaluate an individual's responses to meal combinations and determine if the carbohydrate level needs to be adjusted.

When foods containing simple sugars (concentrated sweets) are included, i.e. desserts, the portion size should be kept to one carbohydrate serving. See the Sweets, Desserts and Other Carbohydrates List in Appendix 11 for exchanges per serving. Many of these foods have traditionally been avoided. Depending upon weight management goals, these foods should be limited if weight loss is desirable. A consistent pattern of carbohydrate is desirable and often achieved in a health care setting, therefore, a regular diet containing regular food is acceptable for diabetes meal planning.

4. **Protein and Fat.** Protein and fat do not affect the blood sugar directly like carbohydrates do. The amount of protein and fat servings do not need to be consistent from day to day since they have little effect on blood glucose levels. The amount of protein and fat that is provided in the General Diet is appropriate for the individual with diabetes in health care institutions.

5. **Exercise.** Most people with diabetes benefit from regular exercise. Exercise improves the body's response to insulin, helps lower blood glucose levels, and is a key factor in the success of clients achieving and maintaining a lower body weight. Individuals using insulin may need adjustments to their meal pattern to prevent hypoglycemia during or after strenuous activity.

6. **Reducing Cardiovascular Risk.** Because the diagnosis of diabetes is a single risk factor for cardiovascular disease, controlling blood lipid levels is an important treatment goal. Advice included in the *Dietary Guidelines for Americans* is especially helpful. However, replacing simple and refined carbohydrate calories with those from monounsaturated fat may be necessary to treat and prevent elevated blood triglyceride for people with diabetes.

7. **Meal Patterns.** Food, exercise, and insulin or oral hypoglycemic agents influence blood glucose concentration. These three influences need to be considered in various ways in the treatment of diabetes. When insulin therapy is used, the activity curve of the insulin determines the times of the day when needs for food are greatest. Exercise reduces the need for insulin and increases the need for food. Usually a regular pattern for taking insulin injections, meals and snacks, and exercise can be worked out so that both hyperglycemia and hypoglycemia can be minimized. This is more important for the person taking insulin.

8. **Measuring Food.** Food should be measured with standard measuring equipment (8-ounce cup, measuring spoons, small food scale, ruler) until the amounts can be estimated accurately. To make certain measurements remain accurate, periodically use measuring equipment to recheck portions served. Foods are measured after they are cooked.

9. **Special Foods.** Special foods are not necessary and may be expensive. Foods labeled "sugar-free," "no sugar," "reduced sugar," or "lower sugar" may be high in fat, calories, and even carbohy-

drates. If these products are used, read nutrition labels carefully. *Sugar-free* does not mean *carbohydrate-free*. However, many sugar-free products are also low calorie and may be used as free foods or aid in weight management goals.

10. **Consistent Carbohydrate Diets in Institutions.** According to the American Dietetics Association position statement (2001), "Providing adequate nutrition is the primary concern for the residents of long-term care facilities if malnutrition is to be prevented or corrected. Experience has shown that residents eat better when they are given less-restrictive diets with regular foods. Therefore, it is appropriate to serve residents with diabetes the regular (unrestricted) menus, with consistent amounts of carbohydrate at meals and snacks. Foods should not be restricted to control blood glucose levels because of the risk of malnutrition."

■ MENU PLANNING

The preferred diet for diabetes is the Consistent Carbohydrate Diet. This implies that the amount of carbohydrates consumed is consistent and the time of the meals and snacks are consistent as well. This pattern will help promote optimal blood sugar control. In most health care settings, acute or long term care, meal times are consistent. The menu can be adjusted to be consistent with carbohydrates for all populations and therefore eliminate therapeutic diets.

Carbohydrate counting is based on choices or grams per meal and snack. The individual is given a carbohydrate allowance that has been individualized to their nutrition therapy and blood sugar goals. One carbohydrate choice equals 15 grams of carbohydrate.

Carbohydrate Choices	Grams of Carbohydrate	Carbohydrate Ranges
1	15	11–20
2	30	26–35
3	45	41–50
4	60	56–65
5	75	71–80

Meal plans may vary from 3–5 choices (45–75 grams) of carbohydrates per meal and 1–2 choices (15–30 grams) of carbohydrates per snacks. Those who use carbohydrate counting to determine the dose of insulin may use a more specific conversion chart.

Conversion Guide	
Total Carbohydrate Grams	**Carbohydrate Choices**
0–5	0
6–10	½
11–20	1
21–25	1½
26–35	2
36–40	2 ½
41–50	3
51–55	3 ½
56–65	4
66–70	4 ½
71–80	5
81–85	5 ½
86–95	6
96–100	6 ½
101–110	7

Carbohydrate allowances may be "spent" at the discretion of the patient; however, not all choices have the same nutritional value and may alter overall nutrition status of the individual. Additionally, frequent poor carbohydrate choices may cause unwanted weight gain and defeat the recommendations for persons with diabetes. The *Exchange Lists for Meal Planning* was prepared by the American Dietetic Association and the American Diabetes Association (see Appendix 11). Use the exchange list for reference in carbohydrate counting.

Snack ideas are outlined as follows:

SNACK IDEAS (Each item equals 1 carbohydrate exchange)

12 animal crackers	8 Townhouse or Ritz crackers	12 mini twist pretzels or 22 sticks
6 frosted animal crackers	1 unfrosted cupcake	4 Starbursts
1 small apple	10-12 Doritos	15 Teddy Grahams
½ banana	½ cup canned fruit	6 vanilla wafers
1" slice banana bread	45-50 Goldfish crackers	⅓ cup low-fat yogurt with fruit
2x2 brownie unfrosted	1 granola bar	2 Oreo cookies
1x2 brownie frosted	15 grapes	2x2 rice crispy
1 "fun size" candy bar	½ cup ice cream	4 wafer cookies
11 candy corn	3 cups popcorn	8 sticks Honey Maid graham crackers
⅔ cup Chex Mix	20 potato chips	1 pouch fruit snacks

Menu portion sizes should be adjusted to reflect goals of nutritional management for individuals in a facility. Patients in acute care settings may be offered a standard diet for diabetes that is consistent in carbohydrate or they may be given a regular menu and the carbohydrate choices may be adjusted based on the carbohydrate allowance for that patient. Traditionally, diabetic diets were ordered as "ADA" with the calorie level indicated. Keep in mind that the American Diabetes Association does not have standard diets nor endorse standardized diets. The term "ADA" diet was attached to calorie levels and over time has been interpreted as a diabetic diet.

The following menu shows an example of adapting a General Diet to a Consistent Carbohydrate Diet providing about 2,000 calories per day.

SUGGESTED MENU PLAN FOR CONSISTENT CARBOHYDRATE DIET

(*Select from foods described*)

MEAL PATTERN	CONSISTENT CARBOHYDRATE DIET	GENERAL DIET
Breakfast 5 carbohydrate choices= ~75 grams carbohydrate	½ cup orange juice (1 choice) ½ cup oatmeal (1 choice) 1 slice toast (1 choice) 1 egg 1 cup milk (1 choice) 1 Tbsp regular jelly (1 choice) 1 tsp margarine coffee	½ cup orange juice ½ cup oatmeal 1 slice toast 1 egg 1 cup milk 1 Tbsp jelly 1 tsp margarine coffee
Lunch or Supper 5 carbohydrate choices = ~75 grams carbohydrate	3 oz roast beef ½ cup mashed potatoes (1 choice) ½ cup broccoli 1 dinner roll (1 choice) 2 tsp margarine 2x2 brownie/frosting (2 choices) 1 cup milk (1 choice) coffee	3 oz roast beef ½ cup mashed potatoes ½ cup broccoli 1 dinner roll 2 tsp margarine 2x2 brownie/frosting 1 cup milk coffee
Dinner 5 carbohydrate choices = ~75 grams carbohydrate	Tuna salad sandwich with 2 slices bread (2 choices) 1 cup tomato soup with 2 crackers (1 choice) ½ cup fruit cocktail (1 choice) 1 cup milk (1 choice) coffee	Tuna salad sandwich 1 cup tomato soup 2 crackers ½ cup fruit cocktail 1 cup milk coffee
Snack 1–2 carbohydrate choices= 15–30 grams carbohydrate	1 cookie (1 choice) 4 oz juice (1 choice)	1 cookie 4 oz juice

■   **GESTATIONAL DIABETES MEAL PLAN**

The meal plan for a woman with gestational diabetes follows the same principles as the Consistent Carbohydrate Diet. The amount of carbohydrates is individualized based on the nutrient needs of the patient. Generally, the meal pattern for breakfast is reduced in carbohydrates due to hormonal surges and insulin resistance in the morning hours. The carbohydrate allowance for breakfast is limited to two choices (30 grams) to help promote optimal blood sugar.

SUGGESTED MENU PLAN FOR GESTATIONAL DIABETES ~2,000 calories

(Select from foods described)

Breakfast: 2 carbohydrate choices (30 grams)

1 slice whole wheat toast (1 choice)
1 egg or 1 tbsp peanut butter
1 tsp margarine
8 oz milk (1 choice)

Snack: 2 carbohydrate choices (30 grams)

3 graham cracker squares (1 choice)
1 Tbsp peanut butter
8 oz milk (1 choice)

Lunch or Supper: 4 carbohydrates (60 grams)

2 slices bread (2 choices)
½ banana (1 choice)
1 cup yogurt (1 choice)
Carrot and celery sticks
2–3 oz protein
2 tsp margarine

Snack: 2 carbohydrate choices (30 grams)

3 cups popcorn (1 choice)
½ cup juice (1 choice)

Dinner: 4 carbohydrates (60 grams)

3 oz chicken breast
1 small baked potato (1 choice)
½ cup broccoli
½ cup peaches (1 choice)
1 small dinner roll (1 choice)
8 oz milk (1 choice)
1 tsp margarine

Snack: 2 carbohydrate choices (30 grams)

6 whole wheat crackers (1 choice)
1 oz cheese
8 oz milk (1 choice)

Once the meal plan is in place, blood sugars are checked on a regular basis. If the blood sugars show a trend of acceptable readings, the meal plan may be adjusted to a higher carbohydrate allowance. This generally does not occur with many gestational diabetics due to hormonal changes during pregnancy. Care must be taken to provide enough calories in the meal plan to promote proper weight gain; extra protein foods at each meal and snack time can aid in meeting calorie needs.

▆ FULL AND CLEAR LIQUID SUBSTITUTIONS

When an individual with diabetes cannot eat solid food, it may be necessary to offer full or clear liquid diets. Carbohydrate counting still plays a role with meal planning. The use of regular products is acceptable to maintain the level of carbohydrate in the meal plan. Sugar-free products should be limited on a liquid diet due to the decreased caloric value. The following table shows carbohydrate values for selected foods that could be offered on a full or clear liquid diet.

Food	Amount	Carbohydrate (grams)	Choices
Carbonated beverages			
Regular soda	1 cup	27	2
Diet soda	1 cup	0	0
Cooked cereal	½ cup	15	1
Creamed soup	1 cup	20	1
Custard, soft	½ cup	18	1
Eggnog, commercial	½ cup	15	1
Flavored gelatin, regular	½ cup	18	1
Ice cream, regular	½ cup	15	1
Light ice cream, vanilla	½ cup	15	1
Sherbet	½ cup	30	2
Sugar	1 tbsp	12	1
Yogurt, flavored low-fat, sugar sweetened	1 cup	40	3

▆ HYPOGLYCEMIA

Hypoglycemia or low blood sugar can be caused by taking too much diabetes medication, eating the wrong amount of carbohydrates at meal time, skipping meals, or getting more exercise than usual. Symptoms may vary among individuals. Common signs are feeling shaky, sweaty, tired, hungry, crabby or confused, rapid heart rate, blurred vision or headaches, and numbness or tingling in the mouth and lips. In severe cases, the person may lose consciousness.

The treatment for low blood sugar is the "Rule of 15." This means once the low blood sugar is known, 15 grams of carbohydrate are given.

TREATMENT OF LOW BLOOD SUGAR "RULE OF 15"

Good Choices	Poor Choices
½ cup fruit juice	Donuts
3 glucose tablets	Ice Cream
½ cup regular soda	Candy Bars
8–10 Lifesavers	Meat
1 small box raisins	Pies, Cakes, Cookies
1 cup skim milk	Milkshakes
1 Tbsp honey	Cheese
1 Tbsp sugar	Nuts

The blood sugar should be rechecked in 15 minutes. If the blood sugar remains low, then retreat with 15 grams of carbohydrate. Recheck the blood sugar again in 15 minutes and repeat as necessary until the blood sugar is within normal limits. If the next meal is more than one hour away, serve a snack consisting of 30 grams of carbohydrate, including a protein source, such as a peanut butter sandwich. If the next meal is less than one hour away, continue to monitor the blood sugar levels until mealtime.

Effective treatment for hypoglycemia in the healthcare setting is essential. Historically the addition of table sugar to juice or other liquids has been used to elevate the blood sugar. This is not recommended as it may over treat the low blood sugar. A high blood sugar may be the result, causing a roller coaster effect. A repeat low blood sugar may occur quickly if not treated properly.

■ HERBAL THERAPY

Herbal therapy is becoming more common to aid in the treatment of disease states. The herbal industry is not regulated by the Food and Drug Administration (FDA) and therefore does not uphold the same standards as other conventional therapies. Persons with diabetes need to exercise extreme caution with herbal therapies, as some may interfere with diabetes medication or may cause the body to become more insulin resistant. Contact a physician or pharmacist for more information.

Additional Resources

American Association of Diabetes Educators. 2001. *A Core Curriculum for Diabetes Education*, 4th ed. Diabetes Management Therapies.

American Diabetes Association. 2005. *All About Diabetes*. Chicago, IL: American Diabetes Assoc.

American Diabetes Association. 2006. Clinical Practice Recommendations. *Diabetes Care*. 29 (Supplement 1).

American Dietetic Association. 2003. *Exchange Lists for Meal Planning*. Prepared by the American Dietetic Association and the American Diabetes Association. Chicago, IL: ADA.

Gifford R, Childs B. 2005. Diabetes Care When You're Sick. *Diabetes Forecast*. Feb:58(2).

International Diabetes Association. 2001. *Gestational Diabetes*. Patient handout.

International Diabetes Association. 2004. *My Meal Plan*. Patient handout.

Jordan M, Hundal RS. 2005. Gestational Diabetes. *Practical Diabetology*. March:24(1).

South Dakota Department of Health Diabetes Prevention and Control Program. 2004. *Diabetes & Herbal Therapy*.

Websites

American Association of Diabetes Educators: www.aadenet.org
American Diabetes Association: www.diabetes.org
Diabetes Care: www.diabetesjournals.org
Diabetes Forecast: www.diabetes.org/diabetes-forecast.jsp
International Diabetes Center: www.parknicollet.com

Study Guide Questions

A. Define and differentiate the following:
   - Type 1 diabetes
   - Type 2 diabetes
   - Gestational diabetes
B. List three factors which can prevent or delay the onset of type 2 diabetes.
C. List at least three goals of nutrition therapy in treating diabetes.
D. List the four main groups of foods which contain carbohydrates.
E. One carbohydrate choice is equal to how many grams of carbohydrate?

F. Using the *Suggested Menu Plan for Consistent Carbohydrate Diet* and the *Exchange Lists for Meal Planning,* plan a full one-day menu for a patient requiring three carbohydrate choices at each meal and one carbohydrate choice snack between each meal and at bedtime. Be sure to include portion sizes.

G. Using the table under *Full and Clear Liquid Substitutions,* plan a full-day menu consisting of four carbohydrate choices (60 grams of carbohydrate) per meal for a diabetic patient on a full liquid diet.

H. List at least four symptoms of hypoglycemia.

I. List at least four good choices for treatment of hypoglycemia.

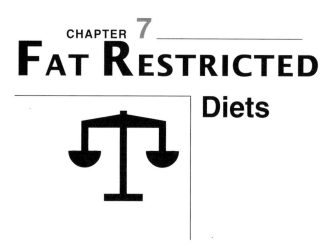

CHAPTER 7
FAT RESTRICTED Diets

Low Fat Diet

(40–50 g fat)

Use

The Low Fat Diet may be prescribed to reduce the fat intake for clients with diseases of the gallbladder, liver, or pancreas, or if disturbances in digestion and absorption of fat occur. For diet management of high blood cholesterol and other blood lipids, see "Cholesterol/ Saturated Fat Restricted Diet" later in this chapter.

Adequacy

The suggested food plan includes foods in amounts that will provide the quantities of nutrients recommended by the National Academy of Sciences for adults. Restriction of fat (the most concentrated source of calories) may result in a diet low in calories. When additional calories are needed, add them in the form of complex carbohydrates. Medium chain triglycerides (MCT) may be useful in meeting energy needs.

Diet Principles

1. The diet is designed to limit fat intake to 40–50 g daily.
2. Foods may cause distress for reasons other than fat content (see "Guidelines for Peptic Ulcer, GERD, Hiatal Hernia" in Chapter 11). If a food is tolerated, it should be allowed.

FOOD FOR THE DAY

	Allowed	Avoid
Milk 3 or more cups	Fat-free (skim) milk, buttermilk made from fat-free milk, fat-free dry milk, non-fat yogurt	Cream, whole milk, low-fat milk (1%) and reduced-fat (2%) milk; ice cream, ice milk; whole milk yogurt, coconut milk
Eggs (if tolerated) Limit to 1 yolk per day including cooking	Soft or hard cooked; scrambled without fat; egg substitutes; egg white as desired	Fried eggs, egg rolls
Meat and Beans 2 servings (4–5 ounces)	Lean beef, pork, lamb, veal, poultry; 95-99% fat-free luncheon meats and hot dogs; fish; cottage cheese, natural or processed cheeses with 5 g or less fat per oz such as part-skim mozzarella, reduced-fat cheddar, or reduced-fat Monterey Jack	Regular luncheon meat, hot dogs, corned beef, sausages, highly spiced, processed meats or fish; fish packed in oil; duck, cuts of pork that are high in fat; all other cheese; peanut butter, nuts
Fruits 1–2½ cups	Any fresh, frozen, dried, or canned fruits; fruit juice	Avocado; any fruit if not tolerated. Any fruit prepared with fat
Vegetables 1–4 cups (including potatoes)	All fresh, frozen, or canned vegetables; vegetable juice; white or sweet potatoes, yams. Any fat used in preparation must be taken from the fat allowance.	Any that may cause discomfort; cabbage family, onion, peppers, sauerkraut, cucumber, dried legumes, rutabagas, turnips, radishes; fried potatoes, potato chips, creamed potatoes
Grains 6 or more servings	Whole-grain or enriched breads, cereals, and grains; whole-grain or enriched macaroni, spaghetti, noodles, or rice; tortillas; plain air-popped or low-fat microwave popcorn; low-fat crackers	Hot breads, such as muffins, croissants, biscuits, waffles, pancakes, popovers, rich rolls, sweet rolls, and doughnuts; party crackers; granola, 100% bran unless well tolerated; fried rice; buttered popcorn
Oils/Fat Limit to 1 tablespoon	Butter, fortified margarine, or salad oil. Use on bread, salads, or in cooking.	
Fluids 6–8 cups	Water and other fluids, such as coffee, tea, fruit or vegetable juice	
Soups	Homemade soups made with fat-free broth or skim milk, with or without allowed vegetable	Commercial soups; soups prepared with cream or whole milk

FOOD FOR THE DAY

	Allowed	Avoid
Sweets/Desserts	Sugar, syrup, and honey; jams, jellies, and preserves; fat-free candy such as jelly beans, marshmallows, and hard candy; cocoa powder and fat-free chocolate syrup Angel food cake; vanilla wafers, graham crackers, gingersnaps; sherbet, fruit ice, non-fat ice cream and frozen yogurt; pudding made with fat-free milk; meringues, gelatin; fat-free commercial baked products	Other cakes, cookies, ice cream, or frozen desserts; pies and pastries; desserts made with whole milk, Whipping cream; cream cheese or egg yolks; chocolate, coconut unless counted in fat allowance.
Seasonings/ Condiments	Vinegar, pickles; ketchup or chili sauce; all herbs and seasonings; white sauce made with skim milk and allowed fat	Olives; cream sauces and gravies unless fat-free

SUGGESTED MENU PLAN FOR LOW FAT DIET

(Select from foods described)

The carbohydrate, protein, fat, and calories will vary depending on whether the smaller or larger amounts of food are served. When fats are restricted, provide additional calories, if needed, through high carbohydrate foods.

Breakfast

Fruit or fruit juice
Cereal/egg
Whole-grain bread
Margarine or butter (1 tsp)*
Skim milk
Hot beverage

Lunch or Supper

Lean meat or substitute (2 oz)
Vegetable
Whole-grain bread
Margarine or butter (1 tsp)*
Fruit
Skim milk

Dinner

Lean meat or substitute (2–3 oz)
Potato, pasta, or grain
Vegetable
Whole-grain bread
Margarine or butter (1 tsp)*

(continued)

Dinner (*continued*)
Fruit
Skim milk

Snacks

Skim milk, fruits, crackers, fresh vegetables

---

*Use on bread or in cooking. Refer to Fat List in Appendix 11, "Exchange Lists for Meal Planning."

Cholesterol/Saturated Fat Restricted Diet

(NCEP/AHA Diet: less than 200 mg cholesterol, 25 to 35% of calories from fat)

Use

The Cholesterol/Saturated Fat Restricted Diet is prescribed to reduce cholesterol and other fatty substances (lipids) in the blood. Current therapy aims to lower LDL (bad) cholesterol and triglycerides and raise HDL (good) cholesterol.

Adequacy

The suggested food plan includes foods in amounts that will provide the quantities of nutrients recommended by the National Academy of Sciences for adults.

Diet Principles

1. Increasing physical activity of all people and weight reduction in overweight patients are effective in improving blood lipid levels.
2. The diet to improve blood lipids (LDL, HDL, triglycerides) follows the Heart Association Guidelines but allows a greater range of fat: 25–35% of total calories.
3. Total saturated fat must stay low, even in higher fat diets. It adds no more than 7% of total calories. (See following table.)
4. When blood triglycerides are high and HDL cholesterol is low, replace simple and refined carbohydrate calories with those from monounsaturated fats to allow up to 35% of total calories from fat. Keep trans fats low (see trans fat table).
5. Complex carbohydrates including whole grains, fruits, and vegetables provide most of the carbohydrates.
6. Reduce dietary cholesterol to no more than 200 mg per day.
7. These diet suggestions may be liberalized for older adults (see "Meeting Nutritional Needs of Older Adults" in Chapter 2). Older adults with high LDL cholesterol levels benefit from the diet

changes listed. Relatively simple modifications to a general diet or liberalized geriatric diet can meet recommendations. These include serving lower-fat milk, avoiding fried foods, gravies and limiting high saturated fat spreads such as butter.

Research has shown that the recent use of statins (cholesterol lowering drugs) in the elderly may not be beneficial and may increase adverse effects such as muscle degeneration and cognitive declines. (*DOC News* July 1, 2005. 12(7) p.10)

8. Additional strategies shown to help lower cardiovascular risk begin with more life-habit interventions (Therapeutic Lifestyle Changes [TLC]).

Diet recommended by the American Heart Association):

- Increase viscous (soluble) fiber foods (such as oat bran and legumes) to 10–25 grams per day.
- Regular, consistent eating of special foods made with plant stanols or sterols (Benecol, Take Control).
- Incorporate at least two servings of fish per week.
- Eat foods high in omega-3 fatty acids: salmon and other fatty fish; canola, soybean, and flaxseed oil; ground flaxseed; and nuts.
- Adjust total caloric intake to maintain desirable body weight.
- Include enough moderate exercise to expend at least 200 kilocalories per day.

MAXIMUM RECOMMENDED GRAMS OF TOTAL FAT AND SATURATED FAT

Daily Calories	Total Fat (25–30% calories) (g)	Saturated Fat (no more than 7% calories) (g)
1500	40–50	12
1800	50–60	14
2000	55–67	15
2200	60–70	17

Common Sources of Trans Fat

Food prepared with partially hydrogenated vegetable oils (baked goods such as cookies, crackers, snack cakes)

Commercially prepared fried foods such as breaded meats, doughnuts

Some margarines

Fried foods served in restaurants and fast food restaurants such as French fries, chicken nuggets, fish patties, fried pies

FOOD FOR THE DAY

	Allowed	Avoid
Milk 3 or more cups	Fat-free (skim) milk, 1% milk, fat-free dry milk, evaporated fat-free milk, buttermilk made from fat-free milk, fat-free soy milk or milk substitutes; fat-free and 1 percent yogurt	Cream, sour cream, whole milk, reduced fat (2%) milk, regular evaporated milk, reduced-fat (2%) or whole milk yogurt
Eggs Limit yolks to 3–4 per week	Hard-cooked, scrambled without fat; egg whites as desired; egg substitutes. Remember to count egg yolks used in cooking toward the total allowed.	Fried egg or egg rolls, unless cooking fat is unsaturated and counted in allowance for day
Meat and Beans 2 servings (total 5–6 ounces)	Lean beef, pork, lamb, veal, poultry; 95–99% fat-free luncheon meats, hot dogs, and sausages; fish; cottage cheese, natural or processed cheeses with 5 g or less fat per oz such as mozzarella, reduced-fat cheddar, or reduced-fat Monterey Jack	Fat beef, pork, lamb, and any visible fat on meat; bacon, salt pork, spareribs, hot dogs, sausage, regular cold cuts, canned meats; skin of chicken or turkey, duck, goose; fish canned in oil; organ meats; cheese other than that allowed, cream cheese
Fruits 1–2½ cups	Any fresh, frozen, dried, or canned fruits; fruit juice, avocado	Coconut
Vegetables 1–4 cups (including potatoes)	All fresh, frozen, or canned vegetables; vegetable juice; white or sweet potatoes, yams. Any fat used in preparation must be taken from the fat allowance.	Commercial fried vegetables, vegetables in butter, cream sauce or cheese sauce, fried potatoes, French fries, chips
Grains 6 or more servings	Whole-grain or enriched breads, cereals, and grains; rice, macaroni; tortillas; Melba toast, matzo bread, bagels, breadsticks, rye wafers, saltines, graham crackers, pretzels, low fat crackers; muffins, biscuits, griddle cakes, waffles made with egg substitute or egg white and allowed fats	Egg noodles; fried rice; commercial muffins, biscuits, doughnuts, sweet rolls, croissants; egg or cheese breads; party crackers; regular granolas, regular granola bars
Oils/Fat 1½ to 3 tablespoons	Vegetable oils; trans-fat free and reduced-fat margarines; low-fat or non-fat salad dressings or those made with vegetable oil; see Fat List in Appendix 11	Butter, ordinary margarine; solid shortening, lard, salt pork, chicken fat, coconut oil, chocolate; creamy salad dressings; nondairy creamers

FOOD FOR THE DAY

	Allowed	Avoid
Fluids 6–8 cups	Water and other fluids, such as coffee, tea, fruit or vegetable juice	
Soups	Homemade soups made with fat-free broth or fat-free milk	Commercial cream soups; soups prepared with cream or whole milk
Sweets/Desserts	Gelatin desserts; angel food cake; low-fat cookies; pies, cake, or cookies made with allowed oils and egg substitute, egg whites, or allowed egg yolks within fat allowance; sherbet, fat-free ice cream or frozen yogurt, light ice cream; commercial low-fat and fat-free cookies, pastries, and desserts; simple puddings prepared with fruit juice or fat-free milk and egg substitute, egg whites, or allowed egg yolks; cocoa (powder not chocolate) Sugar, syrup, honey; jelly and jam; gumdrops, hard candy, jelly beans	Puddings, custards, and ice creams unless made with fat-free milk or fat-free dry milk; whipped cream desserts, whipped toppings; pies, cakes, and cookies unless made with allowed oils and egg yolks; Candies made with chocolate, butter, or cream; commercially prepared popcorn
Seasonings/ Condiments	All spices, seasonings, and flavorings	

SUGGESTED MENU PLAN FOR CHOLESTEROL/SATURATED FAT RESTRICTED DIET

(Select from foods described)

Breakfast

Fruit
Egg (no more than 3–4 yolks per week)
Cereal
Whole-grain bread
Margarine or oil (1–3 tsp)*
Skim milk
Hot beverage

Lunch or Supper

Lean meat or substitute (2–3 oz)
Vegetable
Whole-grain bread
Margarine or oil (1–3 tsp)*
Fruit
Skim milk

(continued)

Dinner (*continued*)

Lean meat or substitute (2–3 oz)
Potato, pasta, or grain
Vegetable
Whole-grain bread
Margarine or oil (1–3 tsp)*
Fruit
Skim milk

*May be used on bread, salads, or in cooking. Refer to Fat List in Appendix 11, "Exchange List for Meal Planning."

Additional Resources

American Heart Association. 2000. Scientific Statement: AHA Dietary Guidelines, revision 2000, #71-0193. *Circulation.* 102: 2284–99.

Krauss, RM et al. 2000. AHA Dietary Guidelines: Revision 2000: A statement for healthcare professionals from the nutrition committee of the American Heart Association. *Stroke.* 31:2751–2766.

Third Report of the NCEP on Detection, Evaluation, and Treatment of High Blood Cholesterol in Adults, National Institutes of Health. 2002. *JAMA.* 106:3143–3421.

Websites

American Heart Association: www.americanheart.org
National Heart, Lung, and Blood Institute's Therapeutic Lifestyle Changes (TLC) diet: www.nhlbi.nih.gov/chd/lifestyles.htm

Study Guide Questions

A. List at least three diseases for which a low fat diet may be prescribed.

B. The Low Fat Diet limits fat consumption to ____–____ grams of fat per day.

C. List at least three common sources of trans fats.

D. The Cholesterol/Saturated Fat Restricted Diet limits cholesterol to less than ____ mg of cholesterol and ____% to ____% of calories from fat.

E. Describe in detail at least three of the eight diet principles presented for the Cholesterol/Saturated Fat Restricted Diet.

F. Modify the general menu planned in Chapter 2 for an individual on a Low Fat Diet. What modifications would you make for a client on a Cholesterol/Saturated Fat Restricted Diet?

CHAPTER **8**

SODIUM RESTRICTED
Diets

No Added Salt Diet

(Low Salt Diet)
(3,000–4,000 mg sodium [130–164 mEq])

Use

The No Added Salt Diet (3,000–4,000 mg sodium) is useful in preventing or controlling edema and/or hypertension. For management of fluid restrictions, see "Fluid Restrictions" in Chapter 9.

Adequacy

The suggested food plan provides foods in amounts that will provide quantities of nutrients recommended by the National Academy of Sciences for adults.

Diet Principles

1. Table salt (which is sodium chloride, containing about 40% sodium) and foods processed with salt are limited. Certain foods that contain liberal amounts of natural sodium and other foods that contain sodium compounds may be limited. The General Diet (including lightly salted foods) is served without a salt packet and with the appropriate restrictions noted.
2. Some medications, including over-the-counter preparations for treatment of indigestion or excess acid, contain large amounts of sodium.
3. Salt substitutes may promote acceptance of sodium-restricted diets but should be used only if permitted by the physician.

FOOD FOR THE DAY	FOOD TO LIMIT (FOOD HIGH IN SODIUM)
Milk 2–3 cups	Buttermilk, instant cocoa mixes
Meat and Beans 2–3 servings (total 2–7 ounce- equivalents)	Smoked, salted, cured, koshered meats or fish such as bacon, bologna, chipped beef, corned beef, hot dogs, ham, luncheon meats, Canadian bacon, pickled meats, salt pork, sausage, anchovies, caviar, pickled herring; regular canned tuna, salmon, sardines; imitation crab or lobster (surimi); processed cheese, cheese spreads, or sauces; most commercial entrees; regular peanut butter in excess of 1 tablespoon per day
Fruits 1–2½ cups	Maraschino cherries, fruits dried with sodium sulfite
Vegetables 1–4 cups (including potatoes)	High sodium packaged potato products; sauerkraut; tomato juice or vegetable juices canned with salt; vegetables seasoned with ham, bacon, or salt pork
Grains 3–10 servings	Breads, rolls, or crackers with salted toppings; pretzels with salt, cheese puffs, corn chips, potato chips; high sodium frozen or packaged rice, macaroni, or noodle mixtures; salted popcorn; instant hot cereals; commercial bread stuffing
Oils/Fat Use sparingly	Salted gravy, bacon, salt pork, seasoned dips, salted nuts, limit salad dressings to 1 tablespoon per day
Fluids 6–8 cups	Commercially canned soups, bouillon, broths, or consommé, dehydrated soup mixes; bouillon cubes, granules, or packets
Seasonings/ Condiments	Any seasoning or combination of seasonings that adds more than 140 mg sodium per serving; salt and salt-based seasonings such as celery salt, garlic salt, onion salt, lemon pepper, seasoned salt, sea salt; meat tenderizer, flavor enhancers (MSG), oyster, black bean and hoisin sauces, meat sauces and cooking sauces, steak sauce, regular soy sauce, teriyaki sauce, barbecue sauce, salsa, ketchup, chili sauce, miso dressing, imitation or real bacon bits, horseradish prepared with salt, most seasoned vinegars; salt substitute, unless approved by physician or dietitian
	Olives, pickles, relishes; salted snack foods such as cheese puffs, corn chips, potato chips, pretzels; high sodium packaged mixes

SUGGESTED MENU PLAN FOR NO ADDED SALT DIET

(3,000–4,000 mg sodium [130–164 mEq])

The suggested menu plan for the General Diet should be used with limitation of the foods listed above, which are high in sodium.

Low Sodium Diet

(2,000 mg sodium [86 mEq])

Use

The Low Sodium Diet (2,000 mg sodium) is useful in preventing or controlling edema and/or hypertension. For management of fluid restrictions, see "Fluid Restrictions" in Chapter 9.

Adequacy

The suggested food plan provides foods in amounts that will provide quantities of nutrients recommended by the National Academy of Sciences for adults. Researchers have found that taking in less than 2,400 milligrams of salt a day was associated with a higher risk of heart disease (JAMA 1999; 282:2068–2070). The DASH diet (Dietary Approaches to Stop Hypertension) principles suggest a combination diet can best control high blood pressure. Maintaining a healthy weight, adding more fruits and vegetables, and eating less saturated and total fat are suggested.

Diet Principles

1. Prepare all foods without salt and do not add salt at the table. Avoid all processed and prepared foods and beverages high in sodium.
2. Limit the amounts of milk, meat, ready-to-eat cereals, and breads and desserts made with salt and baking powder or soda.
3. Some medications, including over-the-counter preparations for treatment of indigestion or excess acid, contain large amounts of sodium.
4. Local water supplies and water that has been chemically softened may contain considerable sodium. The amount of sodium in water should be determined and considered in menu planning.
5. Salt substitutes may promote acceptance of sodium-restricted diets, but should be used only if permitted by physician.

FOOD FOR THE DAY

	Allowed	Avoid
Milk 2–3 cups	Up to 4 cups fat-free (skim), low-fat (1 percent), reduced-fat (2 percent), whole, or chocolate milk per day; 1 cup yogurt may be substituted for 1 cup milk if desired	Commercial cultured buttermilk, instant cocoa mixes, malted milk, milk shakes, milk mixes
Meat and Beans 2–3 servings (total 2–7 ounce-equivalents)	Meat, fish, poultry, eggs, dried beans or peas, prepared or processed without salt; low sodium cheese* or cottage cheese; low sodium peanut butter; boxed, frozen, or canned entrees if less than 500 mg sodium per serving	Meat, fish, poultry, eggs processed or prepared with salt or sodium compounds; koshered meats; smoked salt-cured meats or fish such as bacon, bologna, chipped beef, hot dogs, ham, luncheon meats, pickled meat, salt pork, sausage;

(continued)

FOOD FOR THE DAY *(continued)*

	Allowed	Avoid
		anchovies, caviar, pickled herring, canned tuna, salmon, and sardines; shell fish such as crab, oysters, scallops, and shrimp; imitation crab or lobster (surimi); boxed, frozen, or canned entrees if more than 500 mg sodium per serving; all cheese except low sodium cheese; regular peanut butter
Fruits 1–2½ cups	All fruits and fruit juices	None
Vegetables 1–4 cups (including potatoes)	Fresh, frozen, or unsalted canned vegetables except those listed to avoid; unsalted tomato sauce or paste	Regular salted canned vegetables and vegetable juices, tomato sauce, sauerkraut and other vegetables in brine; frozen vegetables in sauce; canned hominy, frozen, canned or instant potatoes or substitutes to which salt or sodium compounds have been added
Grains 3–10 servings	Regular yeast bread and rolls, up to 4 servings; homemade quick breads including muffins, biscuits, pancakes, and waffles made with regular baking powder or soda; crackers with unsalted tops; rusk; zwieback; Melba toast; unsalted tortilla shells; unsalted rice cakes; cooked enriched and whole-grain cereals and most ready-to eat cereals; whole-grain or enriched macaroni, spaghetti, noodles, or rice prepared without salt; low sodium* or homemade bread crumbs	Bread, rolls, or crackers with salted topping, quick breads; biscuit and quick bread mixes; instant hot cereals, in excess of 1 serving per day; canned, frozen, or prepackaged prepared rice, macaroni, or noodle mixtures; commercial bread stuffing; regular bread or cracker crumbs
Oils/Fat Use sparingly	Regular butter or margarine, salad oil, lard, or vegetable shortening; unsalted gravy; sour cream, low sodium mayonnaise, and salad dressing; low sodium peanut butter; unsalted nuts	Salted or canned gravies, bacon, salt pork, seasoned dips, salted nuts; regular salad dressing and mayonnaise

FOOD FOR THE DAY

	Allowed	Avoid
Sweets/Desserts	Ice cream, sherbet, light ice cream, pudding, or fruit-flavored yogurt when used as part of milk allowance; 1 serving per day of baked dessert made with salt, baking powder, or baking soda; other desserts and sweets made without milk, baking powder or baking soda; sugar and sugar substitutes; jam, jelly, honey, syrup; candy made from allowed foods.	Instant pudding mixes; baked desserts made with salt, baking powder or baking soda in excess of 1 serving per day
Fluids 6–8 cups	Any homemade low sodium* broth or soup made with allowed foods; low sodium* commercial soups or bouillon; coffee, tea or decaffeinated coffee; carbonated beverages	All regular commercial broth, soup, bouillon, consommé (instant, canned or frozen); carbonated beverages containing more than 35 mg of sodium per serving; softened water used for cooking or drinking
Seasonings/ Condiments	Any seasoning that adds 5 mg or less sodium per serving; spices and herbs, lemon juice, vinegar, cocoa powder, unsalted nuts, unsalted popcorn, and unsalted tortilla chips; low sodium* ketchup or mustard, low sodium pretzels or potato chips	Any seasoning or combination of seasonings that adds more than 5 mg sodium per serving; salt and salt-based seasonings such as celery salt, garlic salt, onion salt, lemon pepper, seasoned salt, sea salt; meat tenderizer, flavor enhancers (MSG); meat sauces and cooking sauces, steak sauce, regular soy sauce, teriyaki sauce, Worcestershire sauce, barbecue sauce, salsa, ketchup, chili sauce, imitation or real bacon bits, horseradish prepared with salt, prepared mustard, most seasoned vinegars; salt substitute, unless approved by physician or dietitian
Other		Pickles, olives; relishes; salted snack foods such as popcorn, nuts, corn chips, potato chips, or pretzels

*Low sodium foods contain no more than 140 mg of sodium per serving.

SUGGESTED MENU PLAN FOR LOW SODIUM DIET

(2,000 mg sodium [86 mEq])
(Select from foods described)

Breakfast

Fruit or juice
Cereal with milk and/or egg
Whole-grain bread or toast with margarine or butter, jelly or jam
Hot beverage

Lunch or Supper

Soup or juice, if desired
Meat or meat substitute
Vegetable
Whole-grain bread with margarine or butter
Fruit or allowed desserts
Milk

Dinner

Meat or meat substitute
Potato, pasta, or grain
Vegetable, cooked
Vegetable or fruit salad
Whole-grain bread with margarine or butter
Fruit or allowed desserts
Milk

Websites

National Heart, Lung, and Blood Institute: www.nhlbi.nih.gov/

Study Guide Questions

A. The No Added Salt (Low Salt) Diet limits sodium to between
   ____–____ mg per day.
B. List two conditions which the No Added Salt Diet may help to
   prevent or control.
C. Using the Food for the Day table for the No Added Salt Diet, list
   at least two foods from each food group that should be limited.
D. The Low Sodium Diet limits sodium to ____ mg per day.
E. Modify the general menu planned in Chapter 2 for an individual
   on a No Added Salt Diet. What additional modifications would
   you make for a patient on a Low Sodium Diet?

CHAPTER 9

DIETS FOR
Renal and Liver Disease

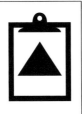

Protein and Electrolyte Controlled Diet

Use

The Protein and Electrolyte Controlled Diet may be prescribed for liver (hepatic) or kidney (renal) disease in which a physician orders specific levels of protein, electrolyte, and/or fluid intakes. Dietary restrictions shall be calculated and taught to the individual or caregiver by a registered dietitian. In keeping with the position of the American Dietetic Association on liberalizing the diet prescription for older adults in long-term care, (8) refer to the Modified Renal Diet later in this chapter.

Adequacy

This diet may not provide adequate quantities of protein, iron, calcium, thiamin, riboflavin, niacin, and vitamin D as recommended by the National Academy of Sciences for adults.

Diet Principles

1. At least half of the total protein should be of high biological value (such as that found in eggs, dairy products, poultry, fish, and meat) with grain, fruit, and vegetables providing the rest of the protein.
2. Adequate caloric intake is essential to ensure protein is used for tissue growth and repair rather than for energy needs. Additional calories may be incorporated through the use of fats; sugar; high-calorie, low-protein formulas; and low-protein bread products. For further information about special products, see *National Renal Diet: Professional Guide*, Chicago: American Dietetic Association, 2002.
3. Fluid limits should be individualized.

4. Salt substitutes (potassium chloride) SHOULD NOT be used unless authorized by a physician. This will affect the potassium level of the total diet.
5. In liver failure, protein, sodium, and fluid restrictions are the usual restrictions.
6. In kidney failure, depending on the stage of kidney disease, any combination of restrictions is possible. Generally, sodium is the first restriction in early kidney disease, followed by protein, potassium, and phosphorus. As patients approach dialysis and urine output decreases, a fluid restriction may be added.
7. Acceptable ranges of calculations for the Protein and Electrolyte Controlled Diet prescriptions are:

Protein   ± *5* G
Sodium   *up to 100 mg over*
Potassium   *up to 100 mg over*
Phosphorus   *up to 100 mg over*
Fluid   *up to 50 mL over*
(Note: 1 mL = 1 cc)

Exchanges for Protein and Electrolyte Controlled Diet

■ MILK GROUP

Milk products are very high in protein, potassium, and phosphorus and are usually limited in the Protein and Electrolyte Controlled Diet. Milk substitutes, such as low potassium liquid nondairy creamers, are frequently used in place of milk.

Milk Products

Milk: Fat-free, low fat, reduced-fat, whole, or chocolate	½ cup
Evaporated milk	¼ cup
Half-and-half or light cream	½ cup
Yogurt, plain or fruit-flavored	½ cup
Ice cream, regular or light	½ cup
Buttermilk, cultured	½ cup
Cream cheese	3 Tbsp
Sour cream	¼ cup

■ MEAT/PROTEIN GROUP

Measure portion size based on meat that is cooked with all the bone and fat removed. Up to 1 out of every 4 ounces of uncooked weight may be lost during cooking.

1 SERVING = 1 OUNCE COOKED MEAT	
Beef	1 oz
Pork	1 oz
Lamb	1 oz
Veal	1 oz
Fish	1 oz
Poultry	1 oz
Cheese*	1 oz
Egg	1 large
Egg whites	2
Egg substitute	¼ cup
Cottage cheese	¼ cup
Peanut butter*	2 Tbsp

*Cheese and peanut butter are high in phosphorus and should be limited to once a week.

Avoid all meats high in sodium as listed in the No Added Salt Diet if the patient is on a sodium restriction. Liver is generally excluded from the Renal Diet because of the high content of phosphorus. Peanut butter is allowed in only small amounts due to phosphorus content.

▪ GRAIN GROUP

Each of the following portions equals one serving. (If portions for diabetics are different from the listed portions, they are shown in parentheses.)

Breads, Cereals, and Grains	
Bread (white is preferred)	1 slice
Hamburger or hot dog bun	½
Rice or pasta (cooked)	½ cup
Cold cereal, refined (no bran)	¾ cup
Puffed rice	1½ cups
Puffed wheat	1 cup
Cream of Rice, Cream of Wheat (cooked)	½ cup
Farina, Malt-O-Meal (cooked)	½ cup
Grits (cooked)	½ cup
Oatmeal (cooked)	⅓ cup
Cornmeal (cooked)	¾ cup
Flour	2½ Tbsp
Donut	1

(continued)

Breads, Cereals, and Grains *(continued)*

Pancake or waffle (1 ounce)	1
English muffin or bagel	½
Flour tortilla (6-in. diameter)	1
Corn tortillas (6-in. diameter)	2
Muffin or biscuit (no nuts or bran)	1
Dinner roll (1 ounce)	1
Pita bread (6-in. diameter)	½
Crackers and Snacks (unsalted)	
Graham crackers	3 squares
Saltines or round butter crackers	4 squares
Melba toast	3 oblongs
Tortilla chips	¾ oz (9)
Pretzel sticks or rings	¾ oz (10)
Popcorn, plain, popped	1½ cups
Desserts	
Vanilla wafers	10 (5)
Cake	2 in. x 2 in.
Angel food cake	1 ounce (1/20 cake)
Cookie (omit 1 fat exchange)	one 3-in. diameter
Sugar wafers	4
Shortbread cookies	4
Sandwich cookies, no chocolate	4
Sugar cookies	4
Fruit pie	⅛
Sweetened gelatin	½ cup
Sherbet	¼ cup

Avoid breads high in sodium as listed in the No Added Salt Diet if the patient is on a sodium restriction. Use whole grains, granola, granola bars, and bran only when advised by a dietitian.

■ VEGETABLE GROUP

Each serving equals ½ cup unless listed otherwise. (If portions for diabetics are different from the listed portions, they are shown in parentheses.)

Low Potassium

Bean sprouts

Cabbage, raw

Cucumbers, peeled
Green beans
Green pepper
Lettuce   1 cup
Wax beans
Chinese cabbage, raw
Chard, raw
Endive
Escarole
Water chestnuts, canned
Watercress

Medium Potassium
Artichoke
Broccoli
Cabbage, cooked
Carrots
Cauliflower
Celery, raw   1 stalk
Collards
Eggplant
Mustard greens
Onions
Radishes
Spinach, raw
Squash, summer
Turnip greens
Turnips
Kale
Sauerkraut (omit 3 salt choices)

The following medium potassium vegetables are high in phosphorus and should be used only with the approval of a dietitian.
Corn   ½ ear (¼ cup)
Mushrooms, canned or fresh raw
Peas   (¼ cup)
Snow peas

High Potassium
Avocado   ¼ whole
Beets
Kohlrabi
Potato, boiled or mashed   (¼ cup)
Pumpkin

(continued)

High Potassium *(continued)*

Tomatoes	1 medium
Tomato juice or vegetable juice cocktail	
(if canned with salt, omit 2 salt choices)	
Tomato puree	2 Tbsp
Tomato sauce	¼ cup

The following vegetables are high in potassium and/or phosphorus and should be used only with the approval of a dietitian.

Asparagus	5 spears
Bamboo shoots, fresh cooked	
Beet greens	¼ cup
Brussels sprouts	
Chard, cooked	
Chinese cabbage, cooked	
Mushrooms, fresh cooked	
Okra	
Parsnips	
Potato, baked	2½ oz
Potato, hashed brown	
Potato chips (omit 1 fat exchange)	1 oz
Rutabagas	
Spinach, cooked	
Sweet potatoes	¼ cup
Winter squash	¼ cup

Avoid all dried beans and peas such as pork and beans, refried beans, split peas, and kidney beans because of their high potassium, protein, and phosphorus contents. Avoid vegetables listed in the No Added Salt Diet if patient is on a sodium-restricted diet. If vegetables canned with salt are used, count each serving as one salt choice.

■ FRUIT/JUICE GROUP

Each serving is ½ cup or one small serving fruit unless listed otherwise. For patients on a fluid restriction, drain canned fruit before serving.

Never give star fruit to a person with kidney disease, as it is toxic to them.

Low Potassium

Applesauce

Blueberries

Cranberries	1 cup
Grape juice	
Lemon	$\frac{1}{2}$
Papaya nectar	
Peach nectar	
Pears, canned	
Pear nectar	
Medium Potassium	
Apple	($2\frac{1}{2}$-in. diameter)
Apple juice	
Apricot nectar	
Blackberries	
Cherries	
Fruit cocktail	
Grapes	15 small
Grapefruit	$\frac{1}{2}$ small
Grapefruit juice	
Lemon juice	
Mandarin oranges	
Mango	
Papaya	
Peaches, canned	
Peach, fresh	(2-in. diameter)
Pineapple, canned or fresh	
Pineapple juice	
Plums	1 medium
Raisins	2 Tbsp
Raspberries	
Rhubarb	
Strawberries	
Tangerine	($2\frac{1}{2}$-in. diameter)
Watermelon	1 cup
High Potassium	
Apricots, dried	5 halves
Apricots, fresh or canned	2 halves
Cantaloupe	$\frac{1}{2}$ cup or $\frac{1}{8}$ small
Dates	$\frac{1}{4}$ cup
Honeydew melon	$\frac{1}{4}$ cup or $\frac{1}{8}$ small
Kiwi	$\frac{1}{2}$ medium
Nectarine	(2-in. diameter)

(continued)

High Potassium *(continued)*

Orange	(2½-in. diameter)
Orange juice	
Pear, fresh	1 medium

The following fruits are very high in potassium and should be used only with the approval of a dietitian.

Banana	½ medium
Prunes, dried or canned	5
Prune juice	⅓ cup

Note: Use 15 g carbohydrate for each serving of unsweetened fruit or juice. Use 25 g carbohydrate for each serving of fruit canned in heavy syrup.

■ FAT GROUP

Unsaturated Fats

Margarine	1 tsp
Reduced calorie margarine	1 Tbsp
Mayonnaise	1 tsp
Low calorie mayonnaise	1 Tbsp
Oil (safflower, sunflower, corn, soybean, olive, peanut, canola)	1 tsp
Salad dressing, mayonnaise-type	2 tsp
Low calorie salad dressing, mayonnaise-type	2 Tbsp
Salad dressing, oil-type	1 Tbsp
Low calorie salad dressing, oil-type	2 Tbsp
Tartar sauce	1½ tsp

Saturated Fats

Butter	1 tsp
Coconut	2 Tbsp
Powdered coffee whitener	1 Tbsp
Solid shortening	1 tsp

Note: Check with the dietitian before using low sodium salad dressing, as many are high in potassium.

■ HIGH CALORIE CHOICES

Use these choices to treat low blood sugar reactions in patients with diabetes.

Beverages

The following are each ½ cup portions:

Cranberry juice cocktail

Lemonade

Limeade

Hawaiian Punch

Kool-Aid

Tang

Carbonated beverages (except those likely to contain potassium and/or phosphorus, including colas, pepper-types, and those containing fruit juice)

Frozen Desserts

Fruit ice	¼ cup
Popsicle	1 bar (3 oz)
Juice bar	1 bar (3 oz)
Sorbet	¼ cup

Candy and Sweets

Butter mints	8
Candy corn	12
Cranberry sauce	2 Tbsp
Gumdrops	9 small
Hard candy	3 pieces
Honey	1 Tbsp
Jam or jelly	1 Tbsp
Jelly beans	6
Lifesavers	8
Marshmallows	3 large
Sugar, brown or white	4 tsp
Sugar, powdered	2 Tbsp
Syrup	1 Tbsp

Avoid chocolate candy, molasses, nuts, and nut butters.

◼ HOT BEVERAGE CHOICES

Coffee, Regular or Decaffeinated	½ cup
Coffee, instant	1 tsp

(continued)

Hot Beverage choices *(continued)*

Cereal grain beverage	½ cup
Instant tea	1 tsp
Tea bag	1
Brewed tea	¾ cup

◼ LOW CALORIE BEVERAGE CHOICES

The following are each ½ cup portions:

Country Time lemonade, sugar-free

Kool-Aid, sugar-free (avoid grape because of high phosphorus content)
Sugar-free carbonated beverages (except colas, pepper-type, and those containing fruit juice)

Tang, sugar-free

◼ SALT CHOICES

Use salt choices only on the recommendation of a dietitian.

Salt	⅛ tsp
Seasoned salts	⅛ tsp
Accent	¼ tsp
Barbecue sauce	2 Tbsp
Bouillon	⅓ cup
Dill pickle	⅙ large or 1½ oz
Mustard	4 tsp
Olives, green	2 medium or ⅓ oz
Olives, black	3 large or 1 oz
Soy sauce	¾ tsp
Light soy sauce	1 tsp
Steak sauce	2½ tsp
Teriyaki sauce	1¼ tsp
Worcestershire sauce	1 Tbsp

The following salt choices are high in potassium and should be used only with the approval of a dietitian:

Ketchup	1½ Tbsp
Chili sauce	1½ Tbsp
Taco sauce or salsa	2 Tbsp

The following foods should be used only with the approval of a physician or dietitian:

Salt substitutes (containing potassium chloride)

Low sodium broth and bouillon (may contain potassium chloride; have dietitian check nutrient analysis before using)

■ FLUIDS

Anything that is fluid or becomes fluid at room temperature counts
as fluid. The following foods count as fluid:

Water
Ice
Juice
Tea and coffee
Pop
Milk
Soup/bouillon/broth
Gelatin
Ice cream/Sherbet
Popsicles

Individuals who require hemodialysis typically have more restrictive
fluid requirements. All liquid consumed, even those with medications, must be counted into the fluid allowance (see "Fluid Restrictions" later in this chapter).

VALUES USED IN CALCULATING PROTEIN AND ELECTROLYTE CONTROLLED DIET

Food Choices	Kcal	Pro (g)	CHO (g)	Fat (g)	Na (mg)	K (mg)	P (mg)
Milk	100	4.0	8	5	80	185	110
Nondairy milk substitute	140	0.5	12	10	40	80	30
Meat	65	7.0	—	4	25	100	65
Starch	80	2.0	15	1	80	35	35
Vegetable							
Low potassium	25	1.0	5	trace	15	70	20
Medium potassium	25	1.0	5	trace	15	150	20
High potassium	25	1.0	5	trace	15	270	20
Fruit							
Low potassium	60*	0.5	15*	—	trace	70	15
Medium potassium	60*	0.5	15*	—	trace	150	15
High potassium	60*	0.5	15*	—	trace	270	15
Oils/Fat	45	—	—	5	55	10	5
High calorie	60	trace	15	—	15	20	5
Hot beverages	trace	—	—	—	—	65	5
Low calorie beverages	trace	—	—	—	—	20	10
Salt choices	—	—	—	—	250	—	—

*Fruits canned in heavy syrup count as 100 calories and 25 g of carbohydrate.
Note: Kcal = calories, Pro = protein, CHO = carbohydrate, Na = sodium, K = potassium,
P = phosphorus.

SAMPLE MEAL PATTERNS FOR PROTEIN AND ELECTROLYTE CONTROLLED DIET			
Protein Level (g)	40	60	80
Calories	1,775	1,800	2,040
Sodium (mg)	1,920	1,845	2,030
Potassium (mg)	2,180 (< 55 mEq)	2,325 (< 60 mEq)	2,860 (< 73 mEq)
Phosphorus (mg)	695	890	1,150
Milk	1	1	2
Nondairy, milk substitute	0	0	0
Meat	3	5	7
Starch	5	8	8
Vegetable	1	1	1
Low potassium	1	1	1
Medium potassium	1	1	2
High potassium	1	1	1
Fruit			
Low potassium	2	1	1
Medium potassium	2	2	2
High potassium	1	1	1
Oils/Fat	9	8	9
High calorie	5	1	0
Hot beverages	2	2	2
Low calorie beverages	0	0	0
Salt choices	3	2	2

Suggested Menus for Protein and Electrolyte Controlled Diet

1,800 CALORIE, 40 g PROTEIN, 2,180 mg (55 mEq) POTASSIUM, 2,000 mg SODIUM, 700 mg PHOSPHORUS DIET	
Meal Pattern	Sample Menu
Breakfast	
1 Medium potassium fruit	½ cup apple juice
1 Starch and 1 salt	⅓ cup salted oatmeal
1 Starch	1 slice toast with
2 Fat	2 tsp margarine
1 High calorie	1 Tbsp jelly
1 Milk	½ cup milk
2 Hot beverages	1 cup coffee

Dinner

2 Meat	2 oz baked fish
1 Starch	½ cup rice
1 Salt and	½ cup salted, cooked
1 High potassium vegetable	spinach
3 Fat	3 tsp margarine
1 Low potassium vegetable	1 cup lettuce salad
1 Fat	1 Tbsp oil-type dressing
1 Medium potassium fruit	½ cup canned pineapple
2 High calorie	1 cup cranberry juice

Lunch or Supper

2 Starch	2 slices white bread for sandwich with
1 Meat	1 oz roast beef
2 Fat	2 tsp mayonnaise
1 Salt and	
1 Medium potassium vegetable	½ cup salted, cooked carrots
1 Fat	1 tsp margarine
1 High potassium fruit	½ cup cantaloupe
1 High calorie	1 popsicle
1 High calorie	½ cup Kool-Aid

Snack

1 Low potassium fruit	½ cup canned pears

1,800 CALORIE, 60 g PROTEIN, 2,325 mg (60 mEq) POTASSIUM, 2,000 mg SODIUM, 900 mg PHOSPHORUS DIET

Meal Pattern	Sample Menu
Breakfast	
1 Medium potassium fruit	½ cup apple juice
1 Starch	⅓ cup oatmeal
1 Meat	1 egg
1 Starch	1 slice toast with
2 Fat	2 tsp margarine
1 High calorie	1 Tbsp jelly
1 Milk	½ cup milk
2 Hot beverages	1 cup coffee
Dinner	
3 Meat	3 oz baked fish
1 Starch	½ cup rice
1 Salt and	½ cup salted, cooked

(continued)

1,800 CALORIE, 60 g PROTEIN, 2,325 mg (60 mEq) POTASSIUM, 2,000 mg SODIUM, 900 mg PHOSPHORUS DIET *(continued)*

1 High potassium vegetable	spinach
1 Starch	1 slice white bread
3 Fat	3 tsp margarine
1 Low potassium vegetable	1 cup lettuce salad
1 Fat	1 Tbsp oil-type dressing
1 Medium potassium fruit	½ cup canned pineapple
Lunch or Supper	
2 Starch	2 slices white bread for sandwich with
1 Meat	1 oz roast beef
1 Fat	1 tsp mayonnaise
1 Salt and	
1 Medium potassium vegetable	½ cup salted, cooked carrots
1 Fat	1 tsp margarine
1 High potassium fruit	½ cup cantaloupe
1 Starch	1 cookie, 3-in.
Snack	
1 Starch	3 squares graham crackers
1 Low potassium fruit	½ cup canned pears

2,000 CALORIE, 80 g PROTEIN, 2,850 mg (75 mEq) POTASSIUM, 2,000 mg SODIUM, 1,150 mg PHOSPHORUS DIET

Meal Pattern	Sample Menu
Breakfast	
1 Medium potassium fruit	½ cup apple juice
1 Starch	⅓ cup oatmeal
1 Meat	1 egg
1 Starch	1 slice toast with
2 Fat	2 tsp margarine
1 Milk	½ cup milk
2 Hot beverages	1 cup coffee
Dinner	
3 Meat	3 oz baked fish
1 Starch	½ cup rice
1 Salt and	½ cup salted, cooked
1 High potassium vegetable	spinach
1 Starch	1 slice white bread

3 Fat	3 tsp margarine
1 Low potassium vegetable	1 cup lettuce salad
1 Fat	1 Tbsp oil-type dressing
1 Medium potassium fruit	½ cup canned pineapple
Lunch or Supper	
2 Starch	2 slices white bread for sandwich with
3 Meat	3 oz roast beef
1 Fat	1 tsp mayonnaise
1 Salt and	
2 Medium potassium vegetables	1 cup salted, cooked carrots
2 Fat	2 tsp margarine
1 High potassium fruit	½ cup cantaloupe
1 Starch	1 cookie, 3-in.
Snack	
1 Starch	3 squares graham crackers
1 Low potassium fruit	½ cup canned pears

Carry-Out Meals and Snacks

People with renal or kidney disease may need to be away from home or their long-term care facility during the day for dialysis or other appointments and treatments. Sending along a midday meal that fits the protein/electrolyte controlled plan will make their day easier and assure ongoing care. Perishable foods should be well-chilled and packed in insulated containers.

Follow the lunch or supper menu plans under "Suggested Menus for Protein and Electrolyte Controlled Diet" earlier in this chapter to create a simple, portable meal:

Sandwich:

Bread, pocket bread, or tortilla

Meat (roasted beef, pork, poultry) with margarine or mayonnaise

or

Egg salad, chicken/turkey salad, or tuna salad

Chef salad and bread/starch:

Cubed meat, tuna, and/or egg with lettuce and acceptable raw vegetables (see below); salad dressing, dinner roll, muffin, crackers, or pretzels

Low or medium potassium fruit:

Small apple, blueberries, grapes, raisins, applesauce, pineapple, or canned, drained fruit such as peaches, pears, fruit cocktail

Low or medium potassium raw vegetable:

Cucumber slices, green pepper strips, lettuce, broccoli, carrots, cauliflower, celery, radishes, turnips

Beverage (regular or sugar-free depending upon diet requirements):

Apple juice, grape juice, cranberry juice cocktail, lemonade, punch,
carbonated beverages including ginger ale, lemon-lime, root beer (no
cola beverages)

Snacks:

To add calories to a meal or for a midmorning or midafternoon snack:

Muffin, bagel with cream cheese, graham crackers, unsalted saltines
or round butter crackers, tortilla chips, unsalted pretzels, vanilla
wafers, animal crackers, approved cookies, sweetened gelatin cup

DO NOT SEND: Bologna, cheese, peanut butter, ham, ham salad, banana, melon, fresh peach, fresh orange, dried fruit, tomato, milk, orange juice, grapefruit juice, tomato juice, cola beverages

Modified Renal Diet

Use

The Modified Renal Diet may be prescribed for individuals with
End-Stage Renal Disease (ESRD) who are on dialysis and reside in a
long-term health care setting. These individuals often have, in con-
junction with other medical conditions, a high incidence of malnutrition, poor appetite, and nausea/vomiting. It is well documented that
individuals who are receiving hemodialysis are often malnourished;
(8) some residents in long-term care with renal disease will not need
a therapeutic diet as a limited appetite precludes the need for restrictions. The use of repetitive, standardized menus in the long-term
health care setting make it possible to individualize the person's nutritional needs based on their biochemistry. The use of the Modified
Renal Diet can allow the person to enjoy the main menu with relatively few changes, a key factor for satisfaction and diet adherence.

The diet principles that follow should be implemented upon initi-
ation of the diet. The facility dietitian and healthcare team will individualize the nutrition therapy as the individual continues with dialysis to maintain adequate calories, protein and fluids according to
laboratory data and renal function. Communication with the renal
clinic about the individual's current progress will provide continuity
of care to promote consistency and the best overall health outcome.
Snacks can be planned to provide additional nutrients without ex-
ceeding restrictions.

Adequacy

The suggested diet plan may not provide adequate quantities of calcium and vitamin D as recommended by the National Academy of Sciences for adults. The Dietary Reference Intake (DRI) for phosphorus and potassium intake may not be met due to the kidney's inability to handle these levels. The dietetic professional will need to recommend appropriate vitamins and minerals as needed.

Diet Principles

The following modifications to the No Added Salt menu provide an example of initial changes in calories, protein, sodium, phosphorus, potassium and/or fluid intakes. The least restrictive menu should be used.

For compliance issues, the practice of providing half-portions of restricted foods is appropriate if these are requested. The dietitian in the renal clinic can also provide recommendations regarding the volume of desired foods that could be consumed either the night before or the morning of dialysis treatments to assist with diet satisfaction.

1. **Energy.** Adequate caloric intake, usually 30–35 kcal/kg, is essential. When calorie intake is inadequate, the body will break down protein for energy instead of using it for essential growth and repair of body tissues.
2. **Carbohydrates.** The addition of refined carbohydrates and simple sugars, i.e. desserts, can be useful in achieving adequate protein-sparing calories.

    If the person with ESRD has diabetes, refer to the Consistent Carbohydrate Diet in Chapter 6. The portion size of simple sugars should be kept to one carbohydrate serving per meal; i.e. a dessert on the menu that equals two carbohydrate exchanges can be served in half the regular portion.
3. **Protein** requirements are higher for persons on dialysis: 1.1–1.4 g/kg on hemodialysis and 1.2–1.5 g/kg on CAPD (Continuous Ambulatory Peritoneal Dialysis). A minimum of 6 ounces of meat or meat alternative should be encouraged. Protein of high biological value is preferable over other protein sources; at least half of the person's protein needs should come from animal sources. Suggestions for increasing protein offered:
    • Double egg portion at breakfast
    • Large portion of meat at midday and evening meal
    • Meat sandwich for snack

4. **Sodium** restrictions will vary according to the patient's hydration status including fluid retention. Sodium may need to be limited to prevent or manage high blood pressure and damaging fluid overload between dialysis treatments. The No Added Salt Diet principles apply along with the following additions:
   - Substitute lower sodium meats to replace high sodium meats as listed in the No Added Salt Diet (see Chapter 8). Either remove the breading on meat, such as that sometimes added to fish and chicken, or select meats with a lower sodium content.
   - Substitute all soup with either appropriately made scratch soups or a low or medium potassium vegetable.
   - Avoid salt substitutes, seasoning mixes, and low sodium broths or bouillons (because of potassium content) unless authorized by physician.
   - Avoid salty snacks.

5. **Phosphorus** needs to be limited and/or treated with phosphate binders to limit bone loss associated with renal disease. The following steps can be initiated to regulate phosphorus intake:
   - Substitute refined carbohydrates (i.e. white bread, Rice Krispies) for whole grain or bran-containing breads and cereals, including oatmeal.
   - Avoid beans and legumes (including pork and beans and baked bean dishes); substitute green beans or other low potassium vegetables.
   - Restrict milk serving to ½ cup per day, preferably whole milk served at breakfast. Frozen yogurt, custard, pudding, and ice cream/ice milk apply to this limitation.
   - Limit cheese intake to ½ ounce per day. (Cream cheese is the exception, as it is low enough in phosphorus to be used without limit.) Cottage cheese (¼–½ cup) and milk-rich desserts are typically not allowed but may be included in a person's nutrition plan upon the discretion of the renal dietitian.

6. **Potassium** plays a role in keeping the heartbeat regular and the muscles working properly. Potassium intake should be individualized as dictated by the person's potassium lab values. Individuals on CAPD (Continuous Ambulatory Peritoneal Dialysis) often experience low levels of potassium and usually do not need a potas-

sium restriction. The following steps can be initiated for a person on hemodialysis:

- Substitute citrus, prune, tomato, and vegetable juices with cranberry, apple, or other low potassium juice (vitamin C-fortified).
- Substitute citrus fruit, bananas, tomatoes, and prunes with low or medium potassium fruits. Fresh tomatoes can be allowed in small amounts (1–2 slices per meal). Star fruit is toxic for the person with kidney disease and should not be served. (43)
- Typically small amounts of tomato sauce are tolerated, i.e. half portion of spaghetti sauce with regular portion of noodles; the meat provided still needs to be a regular or double portion.
- Allow mashed or boiled potatoes if serving size does not exceed ¼ cup per day. Other potatoes, including low salt potato chips, are excluded. No baked potatoes.
- The use of salt substitutes should be restricted.

7. **Fluid** limits, when needed, must be individualized. See the Fluid Restriction section as follows.

Fluid Restrictions

1 oz* = ⅛ Cup = 30 ml = 30 cc	5 oz = ⅝ Cup = 150 ml = 150 cc
2 oz = ¼ Cup = 60 ml = 60 cc	**6 oz = ¾ Cup = 180 ml = 180 cc**
3 oz = ⅜ Cup = 90 ml = 90 cc	7 oz = ⅞ Cup = 210 ml = 210 cc
4 oz = ½ Cup = 120 ml = 120 cc	**8 oz = 1 Cup = 240 ml = 240 cc**

All Foods contain some fluid; however, only foods liquid at room temperature or become liquid when swallowed—like gelatin—need to be counted.

Foods that are considered liquids:

½ Cup Gelatin = ½ Cup fluid = 120 ml = 120 cc

½ Cup Ice Cream or Sherbet = ⅜ Cup fluid = 90 ml = 90 cc

Popsicles (Double) = ⅓ Cup fluid = 80 ml = 80 cc

1 Cup of Crushed Ice = ½ Cup fluid = 120 ml = 120 cc

*oz = Fluid Ounces

SAMPLE MENU PLAN FOR FLUID RESTRICTIONS:

Fluid Restriction	BREAKFAST	LUNCH	DINNER	NURSING and/or SNACKS
1,000 cc (33.3 oz)	240 cc	240 cc	240 cc	280 cc
1,100 cc (36.7 oz)	360 cc	240 cc	240 cc	260 cc
1,200 cc (40 oz)	360 cc	240 cc	240 cc	360 cc
1,300 cc (43.3 oz)	360 cc	360 cc	240 cc	340 cc
1,400 cc (46.7 oz)	360 cc	360 cc	240 cc	440 cc
1,500 cc (50 oz)	360 cc	360 cc	360 cc	420 cc
1,600 cc (53.3 oz)	480 cc	360 cc	360 cc	400 cc
1,700 cc (56.7 oz)	480 cc	360 cc	360 cc	500 cc
1,800 cc (60 oz)	480 cc	480 cc	360 cc	480 cc
1,900 cc (63.3 oz)	480 cc	480 cc	480 cc	460 cc
2,000 cc (66.7 oz)	480 cc	480 cc	480 cc	560 cc

*oz = Fluid Ounces

Additional Resources

Brink BR, Reams SM. 1997. Renal diets for nursing facilities: a team approach. *The Consultant Dietitian.* Consultant Dietitians in Health Care Facilities Practice Group of the American Dietetic Association. 21(4):1, 4–6.

Byham-Gray L, Wiesen K, eds. 2004. *A Clinical Guide to Nutrition Care in Kidney Disease.* Renal Dietitians Dietetic Practice Group of the American Dietetic Association and Council on Renal Nutrition of the National Kidney Foundation. Chicago, IL: ADA-RPG and CRN.

Kopple JD, Massry SG, eds. 1997. *Nutritional Management of Renal Disease.* Baltimore, MD: Williams & Wilkins.

McCann L, ed. 2002. *Pocket Guide to Nutrition Assessment of the Patient with Chronic Kidney Disease,* 3rd ed. New York, NY: National Kidney Foundation.

National Kidney Foundation. 2000. K/DOQI clinical practice guidelines for nutrition in chronic renal failure. *AM J Kidney Dis.* 3(Suppl 2).

Renal Practice Group of the American Dietetic Association. 2002. *National Renal Diet Professional Guide,* 2nd ed. Chicago, IL: ADA-RPG.

Wiggins KL. 2002. *Guidelines for Nutritional Care of Renal Patients,* 3rd ed. Chicago, IL: ADA-RPG.

Wiggins KL. 2004. *Renal Care: Resources and Practical Applications.* Chicago, IL: ADA-RPG.

Study Guide Questions

A. The Protein and Electrolyte Controlled Diet may be prescribed for diseases of the _____ or _____.

B. Who is responsible for calculating and teaching individuals and caregivers about the client's diet restrictions?

C. List at least four sources of high biological value protein.

D. Why is adequate calorie intake essential to individuals on the Protein and Electrolyte Controlled Diet?

E. Milk products are usually limited in the Protein and Electrolyte Controlled Diet because of these three nutrients:

F. Which of the following would NOT be considered a fluid?

    Gelatin
    Ice cream
    Pudding
    Ice
    Popsicles

G. Use of salt substitute, low sodium broth, and bouillon should only be used with the approval of the physician or dietitian. What component of these foods is of particular concern?

H. Plan a sack lunch for a person requiring 3 ounces of high biological protein, 2 starches, 2 fats, 1 low or medium potassium fruit, 1 low or medium potassium vegetable, and 4 ounces of fluid.

I. Plan a full-day menu for a patient on an 80 gram protein, 2,040 calorie, 2,030 mg sodium, 2,860 mg potassium, and 1,150 mg phosphorus diet.

FIBER MODIFIED
Diets

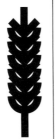

High Fiber Diet

Use

The High Fiber Diet is useful in the treatment of many of the diseases of public health significance—obesity, cardiovascular disease, and type 2 diabetes—as well as the less prevalent but no less significant diagnoses of colonic diverticulosis and constipation. These conditions can be prevented or treated by increasing the amounts and varieties of fiber-containing foods. In addition, a diet higher in fiber is likely to be less calorically dense and lower in fat and added sugar than a diet lower in fiber.

Adequacy

The suggested food plan includes foods in amounts that will provide the quantities of nutrients recommended by the National Academy of Sciences for adults.

Diet Principles

1. The High Fiber Diet contributes 25–30 grams of dietary fiber, defined as plant materials resistant to digestion. Because fiber is found exclusively in plant foods, increase consumption of whole grains (examples: whole wheat, bulgur, oatmeal, whole cornmeal, brown rice, buckwheat, wild rice, whole rye, whole-grain barley, amaranth, millet, quinoa, sorghum, and popcorn), fruits, vegetables, beans, nuts, and seeds. Increased fiber intake should come from a variety of food sources rather than from fiber supplements to ensure adequate nutrient intake.
2. High dietary fiber foods should be added gradually to prevent possible short-term side effects including abdominal discomfort,

bloating, cramping, or diarrhea. If symptoms continue, reduce fiber intake.

3. A high fiber diet should be accompanied by a liberal intake of water or other fluids. Because fiber holds water, thereby softening the stool, at least eight cups of liquids should be ingested daily. Inadequate fluid can lead to constipation or impaction in the colon because dietary fiber absorbs water from the intestinal tract.

4. For patients with diverticulosis, it may be necessary to omit foods such as nuts, popcorn hulls, and sunflower, pumpkin, caraway, and sesame seeds. The seeds in tomatoes, zucchini, cucumbers, strawberries, and raspberries, as well as poppy seeds, are generally considered harmless.

FOOD FOR THE DAY	RECOMMENDED HIGH FIBER FOODS
Meat Average 0 grams fiber/serving **and Beans** Average 5 grams fiber/serving	Cooked dried beans or dried peas, nuts, soybeans, and other legumes. Use whole grains in mixed dishes, such as barley in vegetable soup or stews and bulgur wheat in casseroles or stir-fries. Use whole-grain bread or cracker crumbs in meatloaf.
Fruits Average 2–3 grams fiber/serving	Fruits, especially raw: apples, apricots, bananas, berries, melons, cherries, figs, grapefruit, oranges, peaches, pears, pineapple, plums, prunes, and rhubarb. Skins should be eaten.
Vegetables Average 2–3 grams fiber/serving	Vegetables, especially raw: asparagus, broccoli, Brussels sprouts, carrots, cabbage, cauliflower, celery, corn, green beans, greens, lima beans, okra, onions, parsnips, peas, peppers, potatoes (white or sweet, including skin), radishes, sauerkraut, spinach, squash, tomatoes, yams
Grains Breads & Pasta average 2 grams fiber/serving Cereals average 4 grams fiber/serving	Bran muffins; 100 percent whole-grain breads and crackers listing whole-grain flour as the first ingredient; bran-type and whole-grain cereals; unprocessed bran; use whole-grain flours in cooking whenever possible, substitute whole wheat or oat flour for up to half of the flour in pancake, waffle, muffin or other flour-based recipes; brown rice; whole-wheat pasta
Oils/Fat Nuts average 2–3 grams fiber per ¼ cup	Nuts
Milk 0 grams fiber/serving	None

SUGGESTED MENU PLAN FOR HIGH FIBER DIET

(Select from foods described)

Breakfast

½ cup oatmeal or ¾ cup ready-to-eat whole grain cereal

1 cup skim milk

1 slice whole wheat toast with margarine or butter

1 medium piece of fresh fruit

Lunch or Supper

1 cup chili

2 slices whole wheat bread

2 oz turkey breast

Tomato slice & lettuce leaf

1 medium piece of fresh fruit

1 cup milk

Dinner

3 oz meat

1 medium baked potato with skin

½ cup peas

1 cup lettuce salad with vegetables

Whole-grain bread with margarine or butter

1 cup milk

Snack

1 cup ready-to-eat toasted oat cereal

Low Fiber, Low Residue Diet

Use

The Low Fiber, Low Residue Diet is designed for use in patients receiving radiation therapy on or near the intestine; in partial bowel ob-
struction; in acute gastroenteritis; ulcerative colitis, and diverticulitis;
and in postoperative anal or hemorrhoidal surgery. Long-term use of
this diet is discouraged because it can contribute to constipation, diverticular disease, and colon cancer.

Adequacy

The suggested food plan includes foods in amounts that will provide
the quantities of nutrients recommended by the National Academies
of Sciences for adults, except calcium.

Diet Principles

The diet includes foods that will reduce (not eliminate) the residue in the colon. It is smooth in texture and is mechanically and chemically nonirritating.

Food tolerances vary greatly and clients should be encouraged to eat the most liberal diet possible and include adequate fluids.

FOOD FOR THE DAY

	Allowed	Avoid
Milk Limit to 2 cups	All milk and milk drinks; yogurt. If an individual does not tolerate milk to drink, use in cooking or boil before serving.	Yogurt, if flavored with fruit containing small seeds; milk, yogurt, or foods made with milk in excess of 2 cups.
Meat and Beans 2 servings (total 4–6 ounces)	Ground or well-cooked meat; cottage cheese, mild natural or processed cheese; eggs; smooth peanut butter, if tolerated.	Unless tolerated: spicy meat, fish, poultry; strongly flavored cheeses; cooked dried beans and legumes, chunky peanut butter
Fruits 1–2 cups	Ripe bananas, most cooked or canned fruits	Prune juice; any juice with pulp; most fresh fruits, berries, and other fruit with seeds; dried fruit, raisins
Vegetables 1–4 cups	All vegetable juices, most well cooked or canned without seeds except those listed to avoid; lettuce if tolerated	Corn, peas, spinach, potato skin, winter squash, artichoke, sauerkraut, tomatoes, broccoli, Brussels sprouts, cabbage, onions, cucumbers
Grains 3–10 servings	Enriched white, wheat, rye bread without seeds; cornbread, biscuits, muffins, pancakes, waffles, plain sweet roll; graham crackers made with refined flours, saltines, rusk, zwieback, Melba toast; enriched, cooked refined cereals, such as farina, Cream of Wheat, cornmeal, Malt-O-Meal, strained oatmeal; dry cereals such as puffed rice, riceflakes, cornflakes; spaghetti, macaroni, noodles, or white rice.	Bread, crackers, or cereals containing whole grains, bran, dried fruits, nuts, or seeds; brown or wild rice.
Fats Use sparingly	Salad oils, fortified margarine, butter, cream, mayonnaise, mildly seasoned salad dressings; crisp bacon; plain gravies	Spicy salad dressings, olives, high-fat gravies and sauces

FOOD FOR THE DAY

	Allowed	Avoid
Fluids 6–8 cups	Water and other fluids, such as coffee, tea, fruit or vegetable juice, carbonated beverages	Prune juice, any juice with pulp
Sweets/Desserts	Pudding, custard, flavored or frozen yogurt with allowed fruits (within 2 cup milk limit), gelatin, plain sherbet, fruit ice, popsicles; plain cake and cookies; pie made with allowed fruits; honey, syrups, hard candy, marshmallows; jelly	All desserts and candy containing coconut, nuts, seeds, or dried fruit; jams and preserves
Soup	Cream soups made with allowed vegetables, noodles, rice, or flour; broth or bouillon	All others
Others	Salt, pepper, ketchup, mustard, spices and herbs, vinegar	Nuts and seeds, coconut, popcorn, pickles and relish with seeds

Additional Resources/Websites

National Digestive Diseases Information (NDDIC): http://digestive.niddk.nih.gov/ddiseases/pubs/diverticulosis/index.htm#5

Position of the American Dietetic Association: Health Implications of Dietary Fiber. 2002. *J Am Diet Assoc.* 102: 99–1000 (Expires 2007).

Study Guide Questions

A. List at least three diseases for which a high fiber diet may be useful.

B. The High Fiber Diet contributes _____–_____ grams of dietary fiber.

C. Fiber should be added gradually to prevent what four short term side effects?

D. What are the potential complications of inadequate fluid intake?

E. Long term use of the Low Fiber, Low Residue Diet is discouraged because it can contribute to _____, _____, and _____.

F. Modify the general menu planned in Chapter 2 to include increased fiber foods.

CHAPTER 11

OTHER MODIFIED
Diets

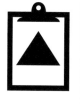

High Nutrient Diet

Use

The High Calorie, High Protein Diet is prescribed for nutritional rehabilitation of the patient following a debilitating disease, surgery, or healing of pressure sores. It is also useful for the prevention of malnutrition in patients who are unable or unwilling to consume adequate nutrients due to cognitive impairment, lack of appetite, or inability to eat normal portions of food. Food choices are made from the General Diet.

Adequacy

The suggested food plan includes foods in amounts that will provide calories, protein, minerals, and vitamins in amounts greater than recommended by the National Academy of Sciences for adults.

Diet Principles

1. Lack of appetite is often a factor for a patient in need of this diet. Careful evaluation of the factors contributing to poor food intake is critical for proper care. Overall quality of food served, food texture, need for assistive devices for self-feeding, and body positioning should be considered.
2. Adequate nutrients are essential for improving skin integrity and healing incisions and pressure sores. Include vitamin C-rich foods at each meal and encourage the eating of foods high in zinc. See list of sources of vitamin C in Chapter 1 and zinc sources in Appendix 9. Protein requirements range from 0.8 to 1.5 grams per kilogram depending on the stage of the pressure ulcer or type of wound and other individual factors. Nutrition supplements and/or

vitamin/mineral supplements may be indicated. Refer to a registered dietitian to assess the nutrient needs for healing.

3. Generally, a patient cannot begin to eat a high calorie diet immediately. Initially, portion sizes may need to be kept small. Increase size and number of servings gradually.

4. Breakfast is often the best-eaten meal of the day and offers an opportunity to increase nutrient and calorie intake. Some individuals eat better if food for the day is served as three small meals with three between-meal snacks. For other patients, a decrease in the number of feedings per day may result in a better appetite and increase total food consumption. Patients' individual differences must be considered.

5. Increase calorie intake mainly from high nutrient foods. Rich pastries, desserts, candy, and fried foods add calories but may decrease patients' appetites for other nutritious foods. Such foods will not add protein or other nutrients that may be needed.

6. A simple addition to each meal may answer the need for increased calories, protein, and vitamins without increasing portion size. For example, serve half and half on cereal; serve extra butter or margarine with cereals, vegetables, and breads; offer "super cereal;" serve an extra glass of milk or a bedtime snack of cereal with milk or cream and sugar; and serve breads with both jelly and margarine or butter.

7. If additional protein is needed within a limited volume or calorie level, non-fat dry milk added to a variety of foods is an effective way of increasing protein. It can be added to fluid milk or to prepared dishes, such as meat loaf or mashed potatoes. The addition of $1\frac{1}{3}$ cups fat-free dry milk to 1 quart of milk will double the protein content.

8. Cream soups will add more calories and protein than broth soups. Adding non-fat dry milk to cream soups further increases their nutritional value.

9. With heavy, high protein, high calorie meals, it may be better to serve a simple dessert such as fruit, pudding, ice cream, gelatin, or cookies.

10. Commercially prepared nutrient supplement products may be used between meals or may be added to liquids and foods for added nourishment and calories. There are a variety of concentrated calorie and protein liquids and powders that can be added to foods and beverages. For older adults, it is recommended that liquid supplements be served at least one hour prior to a meal and not with meals.

SUGGESTED MENU PLAN FOR HIGH NUTRIENT DIET

2,800 CALORIES, 130 g PROTEIN

(Select from foods described)

Breakfast

½ cup fruit or juice

1 egg

½ cup whole-grain cereal

1 slice whole-grain toast with margarine or butter and jelly

1 cup whole milk

Hot beverage

Midmorning

½ cup fortified beverage or nutrition supplement

Lunch or Supper

3 ounces meat or substitute

½ cup vegetable—raw or cooked

2 slices whole-grain bread with margarine or butter

½ cup fresh fruit

1 cup whole milk

Midafternoon

½ peanut butter sandwich

1 cup whole milk

Dinner

3 ounces meat, fish, or poultry

½ cup potato, pasta, or grain with margarine or butter

½ cup cooked vegetable with margarine or butter

½ cup salad—vegetable or fruit with salad dressing

1 slice whole-grain bread with margarine or butter and jelly

Dessert

1 cup whole milk

Bedtime

1–2 oz cheese

6 saltine crackers

1 cup whole milk

Additional Resources/Websites

ADA diet manual, High calorie, high protein diet.

The Council for Nutritional Clinical Strategies in Long-Term Care. 2004. Appetite Problems in Nursing Home Residents: Prevention, Recognition, and Treatment Strategies. April.

Juric A, Gordon KL, Craig LD, Ataya DG. 1998. Nutrition supplementation enables elderly residents to meet or exceed RDA's without displacing energy or nutritional intake from meals. *J Am Diet Assoc.* 98:1457–59.

Kayser-Jones J. 2000. Improving the Nutritional Care of Nursing Home Residents. *Long Term Care Management.* 10:56–59

Litchford, M. 2004. *The Advanced Practitioner's Guide to Nutrition & Wounds and Practical Applications in Laboratory Assessment of Nutritional Status.* Greensboro, NC: CASE Software.

National Pressure Ulcer Advisory Panel: www.npuap.org/biblio.html

Finger Food Modification Diet

Use

The Finger Food Modification Diet is intended for people with Alzheimer's disease, other dementia or cognitive impairment, or certain neuromuscular disorders.

Adequacy

The diet, if carefully chosen from suggested foods, is adequate in all nutrients recommended by the National Academy of Sciences for adults. The General Diet should form the basis of this diet, with only such modifications as to prompt self-feeding and promote independence.

Diet Principles

1. Individuals who resist being fed, are combative, or have difficulty manipulating utensils may increase their caloric intake and stabilize their weight if presented with most of their food in finger food form.
2. Individuals may benefit from this eating approach to decrease frustration, enhance dignity and self-esteem, and increase morale and motivation. Improvement in appetite may also occur.
3. The individual's acceptance of finger foods may determine the appropriateness in relation to dignity.
4. The implied invitation to self-feeding may be responded to by greater mobility in otherwise inert individuals, resulting in enhanced strength and coordination and expanded range of motion.
5. Foods offered should be calorie- and nutrient-dense and should be good sources of fiber.
6. Pacing and restlessness in some clients may elevate energy expenditure beyond that estimated by conventional calculation.

7. An adequate fluid intake should be encouraged. Ample opportunities to drink liquids should be provided.
8. Individuals on consistency altered diets will need further modifications to some of the suggested foods listed below.

■ TIPS

The use of adaptive equipment such as plate stabilizers, plate guards, weighted utensils, rocking knives, nosey cups, spouted cups, and cups or mugs with handles may be useful in certain instances. Cutting foods such as meats, cheese, fruits, and vegetables into strips or wedges provides a "handle" on foods that allows easy self-feeding. Foods cut into bite-size cubes are easy to pick up with the fingers. An occupational therapist consultation may prove beneficial.

FOOD FOR THE DAY	FINGER FOOD SUGGESTIONS
Milk 2–3 cups	Any fluid milk (may be served in mugs), cheese sticks, cubes, or slices, custard pie
Meat and Beans 2–3 servings (total 2–7 ounce-equivalents)	Meat loaf, patties, cutlets, nuggets, tender cut-up meat, fish, fish sticks, sausage, luncheon meats, omelets, deviled eggs, firmly cooked eggs, foods that can easily be made into sandwiches
Fruits 1–2 ½ cups	Cut-up fresh fruits, grapes, drained chunk canned fruits, dried fruit, fruit molded in firm gelatin
Vegetables 1–4 cups	Bite-size cooked vegetables, baked or steamed potatoes, timbales and soufflés, relishes (if adequate dentition), cherry tomatoes
Grains 3–10 servings	Breads, buns, muffins, biscuits, crackers, pita bread, tortillas, pancakes, French toast, bite-size dry cereal without milk, cooked cereal with milk served in a mug, cereal bars, granola bars
Oils/Fat	Nuts, peanut butter, table spreads, salad dressings, mayonnaise, sweet or sour cream, creamers and toppings, applied as appropriate before serving Gravies and sauces can be served in a side dish for dipping
Soups	Strained or blended soups served in a mug
Sweets/Desserts	Cookies, cake, donuts, turnovers, bar cookies, ice cream bars, ice cream sandwiches, finger gelatin, pudding served in ice cream cone
Fluids	Any (may be served in mugs)

SUGGESTED MENU PLAN FOR FINGER FOOD DIET

(Select from foods described)

Breakfast

Fruit juice

Orange sections

Bite-size frosted shredded wheat

Omelet or sausage link

Toast with peanut butter and jelly, quartered

Milk or cocoa

Lunch or Supper

Meat loaf, cubed

Parslied buttered potato, cut up

Fingerling carrots

Firm-molded applesauce in gelatin, cubed

Buttered bran or corn muffin

Oatmeal raisin cookie

Milk

Dinner

Grilled turkey and cheese sandwich, quartered

Cream of tomato soup, in mug

Baked corn custard, firm, cut up

Banana wheels and canned peach slices

Hot beverage

Snack

Apple wedges

Cheese cubes

Additional Resources/Websites

Alzheimer's Association. Eating Fact Sheet. Oct 2004. www.alz.org

Curfman, S. 2005. Managing Dysphagia in Residents with Dementia. *Nursing Homes Magazine*. Sept:1–7.

Dorner, B. General guidelines for serving the finger food diet. Available at: www.BeckyDorner.com

Dorner, B. 2003. I haven't had a thing to eat all day. . . Nutrition for the dementia resident. Available at: www.BeckyDorner.com

Walker, G. 2001. The hows and whys of a finger food diet. *Gerontological Nutrition Newsletter*. Summer:9–12.

Vegetarian Diets

Use

Individuals wishing to avoid foods containing animal products may request a Vegetarian Diet. The Vegan or Total Vegetarian Diet is designed for individuals who wish to exclude all animal products. The Lacto-Vegetarian Diet is designed for individuals who wish to consume plant foods, cheese, and other dairy products. The Ovo-Lacto-Vegetarian Diet includes the addition of eggs. The Semi-Vegetarian Diet is designed for individuals who wish to exclude red meat but include chicken and fish with plant foods, dairy products, and eggs.

Adequacy

The suggested food plans include foods in amounts that will provide the quantities of nutrients recommended by the National Academy of Sciences for adults. The diet requires additional modifications to meet nutritional needs during illness, pregnancy, lactation, infancy, and childhood.

Diet Principles

1. Obtain an accurate diet history; it is essential in determining limitations.
2. Provide adequate nutrients by including mostly foods rich in nutrients and only small amounts of low-nutrient sweets and fats.
3. Limit highly processed grains and other refined carbohydrates to ensure adequate intake of trace nutrients.
4. Avoid excess cholesterol intake by limiting eggs to three or four egg yolks a week for those who consume eggs.
5. Careful consideration should be given to the following when planning vegetarian diets:
   a. **Carbohydrates.** If all animal products are excluded, diets tend to be low in fat and high in dietary fiber. Enough carbohydrate for energy must be provided to allow dietary protein to be used for maintenance and repair and not to meet energy needs, particularly for vegans.
   b. **Protein**. Plant proteins alone can provide enough amino acids (the building blocks of protein) when a variety of plant proteins are eaten throughout the day and the total caloric intake meets the individual's caloric needs. It is no longer recommended that complementary proteins be eaten at the same meal. Substitutes for 1 ounce of meat are:

8 ounces soy milk
½ cup cooked dry beans
2 tablespoons peanut butter
2 tablespoons nuts or seeds
4 ounces tofu or tempeh
1 whole egg or 2 egg whites

c. **Calcium**. Calcium intakes lower than that recommended by the National Academy of Sciences do not seem to cause health problems for vegetarians as long as vitamin D intake or exposure to sunlight is adequate. Vegetarians can absorb and retain more calcium from foods than those who are not vegetarian. See "Calcium Content of Selected Foods" in Appendix 8 for non-animal sources of calcium.

d. **Vitamin D.** Vegans who have limited exposure to sunlight may require vitamin D supplements.

e. **Iron**. Iron in plants is not as readily absorbed as that in meats. To increase iron absorption, include foods rich in vitamin C in the same meal with iron-containing foods. Tea (from tea leaves, not herbal blends) interferes with iron absorption and should be limited. See "Iron Content of Selected Foods" in Appendix 10 for good sources of iron.

f. **Vitamin B-12**. Only animal products contain vitamin B-12. Diets of vegetarians who eat dairy products and eggs are rarely deficient in vitamin B-12. Vegans need a reliable source of vitamin B-12; good fortified sources include fortified cereals, fortified soy beverages, some brands of nutritional (brewer's) yeast, and vitamin supplements.

g. **Zinc**. The absorption of zinc is decreased by dietary fiber, oxalates and phytic acid (common in vegetables and grains), and soy protein, although vegetarians usually have adequate zinc status. See "Zinc Content of Selected Foods" in Appendix 9.

6. Read product labels carefully to avoid hidden ingredients such as meat extracts, animal fats, eggs, and milk.

The following guidelines are for the Lacto-Ovo-Vegetarian Diet. Items marked with an asterisk would be omitted from a vegan (no animal products) meal plan.

FOOD FOR THE DAY

	Allowed	Avoid
Milk up to 3 servings	Fat-free (skim)*, low-fat (1%)*, or reduced-fat (2%)* milk; low-fat flavored or plain yogurt*, low-fat cheese*	Whole milk*, chocolate milk*
Meat and Beans 2–3 servings (total 2–7 ounce- equivalents)	Eggs*, meat analogues, tofu, or tempeh; legumes; soy milk; limited amounts of nuts and nut butters including peanut butter	High-fat cheese*, refried beans
Fruits 1 ½ cups or more	Any fresh, canned, frozen, dried; 100% fruit calcium-fortified orange juice	Avocado
Vegetables 2 cups or more	Any fresh, canned, frozen; tomato juice or vegetable juice cocktail	Deep-fried or battered and fried vegetables
Oils/Fat use sparingly	Margarine, salad dressings, and vegetable oils	Butter*, sour cream*, cream cheese*, nondairy creamers containing coconut oil
Sweets/Desserts use sparingly	Low-fat, moderately sweetened such as pudding/custard made with fat-free milk*, angel food cake*, graham crackers, vanilla wafers, flavored yogurt*, light ice cream*, frozen yogurt*	High sugar, high-fat desserts such as pie and pastries, frosted cake, candy, whole-milk puddings* and custards*, ice cream*
Fluids 6–8 cups	Water, bottled and sparkling waters, coffee, herbal tea	Tea (with meals); carbonated beverages and sweetened flavored, sparkling waters; fruit beverages, drinks and "ades"; beverages containing alcohol
Other	Vegetable broth, herbs and spices, low sodium seasonings, black strap molasses, brewer's yeast, wheat germ	Honey, jelly, and jam; high sodium seasonings

*These items would be omitted from a vegan (no animal products) meal plan.

SUGGESTED MENU PLAN FOR LACTO-OVO VEGETARIAN DIET

(Select from foods described)

Breakfast

Citrus fruit or

¾ cup 100% fruit juice

1 cup whole-grain or enriched cereal

1 cup milk

2 slices whole-wheat toast or other bread with margarine

Lunch or Supper

1 serving meat substitute

1 cup cooked vegetable or

2 cups salad greens

Whole-grain roll or 2 pieces other whole-grain bread

Fruit

1 cup milk or yogurt

(Example: ½ oz low-fat cheese and ¼ cup seasoned pinto beans served over 2 cups of mixed salad greens and raw spinach with salsa; 2 warm corn tortillas; mixed fruit salad with banana and apple; 1 cup skim milk)

Dinner

1 serving meat substitute

1 cup potato, pasta, or grain

1 cup cooked vegetable

Vegetable or fruit salad

Fruit or light dessert

1 cup milk or other beverage

(Example: 4 oz crumbled tofu with 1 cup stir-fried vegetables; 1 cup brown rice; ½ cup carrot, apple, and raisin salad; ½ cup fruit cocktail in juice; 8 oz low-fat flavored yogurt)

Snack

Low-fat yogurt with fresh fruit or

Low-fat whole-grain crackers with low-fat cheese

SUGGESTED MENU PLAN FOR VEGAN VEGETARIAN DIET

(Select from foods described)

Breakfast

Citrus fruit or 100% fruit juice

Whole-grain or enriched cereal with fortified soy milk

2 slices whole-wheat toast or other bread with margarine

Lunch or Supper

1 serving meat substitute

1 cup cooked vegetable or

2 cups salad greens

Whole-grain roll or 2 pieces other whole-grain bread

Fruit

Fortified soy milk

(Example: ½ cup seasoned pinto beans served over 2 cups of mixed salad greens and raw spinach with salsa; 2 warm corn tortillas; mixed fruit salad with banana and apple; 1 cup fortified soy milk)

Dinner

1–2 servings meat substitute

Potato, pasta, or grain

1 cup cooked vegetable

Vegetable or fruit salad

Fruit or light dessert

Fortified soy milk or other beverage

(Example: 4 oz crumbled tofu with 1 cup stir-fried vegetables; 1 cup brown rice; 1 cup cooked broccoli; ½ cup carrot, apple, and raisin salad; ½ cup fruit cocktail in juice; 4 graham crackers)

Snack

Whole-grain bread or crackers

Fresh fruit or protein equivalent

(Examples: Whole-grain bagel with margarine and jelly; fresh pear; low-fat whole-grain crackers with 2 Tbsp peanut butter)

Additional Resources/Websites

American Dietetic Association. 1992. *Eating Well: The Vegetarian Way*. Chicago, IL: ADA.

American Dietetic Association. 1996. *Being Vegetarian*. Chicago, IL: ADA.

Havala, Suzanne. 2001. *Vegetarian Cooking for Dummies*. New York: Hungry Minds, Inc.

Ornish, Dean. 1995. *Dean Ornish's Program for Reversing Heart Disease*. New York: Ballatine Books.

Vegetarian Resource Group: www.vrg.org

Wasserman, Debra and Mangels, Reed. 1999. *Simply Vegan: Quick Vegetarian Meals*, 3rd ed.

Food Allergies and Intolerances

If someone has an unpleasant reaction to something they ate, they might wonder if they have a food allergy. Food allergies affect up to 6 to 8 percent of children under the age of three and 2 percent of adults. One out of three people either believe they have a food allergy or modify their or their family's diet. Food allergy is commonly suspected, yet health care providers diagnose it less frequently than most people believe. In many cases, it is a food intolerance—not a true allergy—that is causing the problem.

Food Allergy

A food allergy is an abnormal response to a food triggered by the body's immune system. It causes the body to produce antibodies called immunoglobulin E (IgE) to fight it. Symptoms may be immediate or delayed up to a few hours, and range from uncomfortable (hives, stomach upset) to life threatening (swelling of the tongue, closing of the throat). A severe type of reaction is called anaphylaxis, commonly known as anaphylactic shock. Anaphylactic shock can produce symptoms such as those listed above in addition to a drop in blood pressure, unconsciousness, and even death. Diagnosis of a food allergy can usually be made based on skin or lab tests and a detailed diet history. If a severe food allergy exists, an antihistamine or epinephrine kit (i.e. EpiPen) should be on hand per medical prescription.

Food Intolerance

A food intolerance is when eating a certain food or foods triggers a negative physiological response, but the immune system is not affected in the same way. Symptoms may take up to three days to show, making food intolerances very difficult to diagnose. Lactose intolerance and gluten sensitive enteropathy (celiac disease) are forms of food intolerances. Elimination diets, detailed diet history, and specialty tests are the most common methods for diagnosis. This is not life threatening, but symptoms may be severe and range from gastrointestinal distress, headaches, and sinus and/or respiratory problems.

Common Food Allergies

In adults, the most common foods that cause allergic reactions are shellfish (such as crayfish, lobster, shrimp, and crab), peanuts, tree nuts, fish, and eggs. The most common foods that cause problems in children are eggs, milk, and peanuts. Presently there are no medications that cure food allergies or food intolerances. Strict avoidance of the allergy-causing food is the only way to avoid a reaction. Reading ingredient labels for all foods is the key to maintaining control over the allergy.

■ MILK ALLERGY

Eliminating all milk and milk by-products from the diet is necessary. This includes yogurt, butter, most margarines, cheese, cream, and milk.

Milk is an important source of calcium, vitamin A, vitamin D, riboflavin, pantothenic acid, and phosphorus. Enriched soy, potato, or rice milk beverages are good alternative sources of calcium, vitamin A, and vitamin D. These enriched beverages can also be used as a substitute for milk in recipes. Alternative sources of riboflavin, pantothenic acid, and phosphorus are found in legumes (such as peas, beans, or soy), nuts, and whole grains.

Reading food labels is crucial. For a milk-free diet, you should avoid foods with these ingredients:

Artificial butter flavor

Butter, butter fat, butter oil

Buttermilk

Casein

Caseinates (such as ammonium, calcium, magnesium, potassium, or sodium caseinate)

Cheese

Cottage cheese

Cream

Curds

Custard

Ghee

Half & half

Hydrolysates (listed as casein, milk protein, protein, whey, or whey protein hydrolysate)

Lactalbumin, lactalbumin phosphate

Lactoglobulin

Lactose

Lactulose

Milk (derivative, powder, protein, solids, malted, condensed, evaporated, dry, whole, low-fat, non-fat, skimmed, and goat's milk)

Nougat

Pudding

Rennet casein

Sour cream, sour cream solids

Sour milk solids

Whey (in all forms, including sweet, delactosed, and protein concentrate)

Yogurt

◼ EGG ALLERGY

Eggs must be avoided completely, even if a diagnosis of allergy to only egg whites or egg yolks has been made. It is very difficult to separate the egg white and yolk from each other completely, without having some cross contamination. Eggs provide the diet with vitamin B-12, pantothenic acid, folate, riboflavin, selenium, and biotin. These nutrients can be easily provided by other foods in the diet, such as whole grains, legumes, and meat products.

Reading food labels is crucial. For an egg-free diet, you should avoid foods with these ingredients:

Albumin

Egg (white, yolk, dried, powdered, solids)

Egg substitutes

Eggnog

Globulin

Livetin

Mayonnaise

Meringue

Ovalbumin

Ovomucin

Ovomucoid

Ovovitellin

◼ PEANUT ALLERGY

Peanuts and peanut derivatives need to be avoided. Peanuts provide niacin, vitamin E, magnesium, chromium, and manganese. A diet with a variety of vegetables, whole grains, meats, and legumes will meet these needs as well.

Reading food labels is crucial. For a peanut-free diet, you should avoid foods with these ingredients:

Beer nuts

Peanut oil

Ground nuts

Mixed nuts

Peanuts

Peanut butter

Peanut flour

▪ TREE NUT ALLERGY

An allergy to tree nuts is one of the most common food allergies in adults. Tree nuts include almonds, brazil nuts, cashews, chestnuts, hazelnuts, hickory nuts, pecans, pine nuts, pistachios, walnuts, and macadamia nuts.

Tree nuts are being added to many foods, so reading food labels is very critical with this food allergy. For a tree nut-free diet, you should avoid foods with these ingredients:

Almonds

Brazil nuts

Cashews

Chestnuts

Filbert/hazelnuts

Gianduja (creamy mixture of chocolate and chopped toasted nuts found in premium or imported chocolate)

Hickory nuts

Macadamia nuts

Almond paste

Mashuga nuts

Nougat

Nu-Nuts artificial nuts

Nut butters

Nut meal

Nut oil

Nut paste (such as almond paste)

Pecans

Pine nuts

Pistachios

Walnuts

▪ FISH AND SHELLFISH ALLERGIES

All species of fish should be avoided if diagnosed with a fish allergy. For a shellfish allergy, shrimp, crabs, lobster, and crawfish, and mollusks, such as clams, oysters, and scallops, should be avoided.

Foods that contain fish or fish products are Worcestershire sauce (if it contains anchovy), Caesar salad, caviar, and roe (fish eggs). Surimi is made from fish muscle that is reshaped and used to make imitation seafood (like imitation crab legs, crab cakes, and imitation lobster products).

Nutrients that are found in fish can also be found in meats, grains, legumes, and oils, therefore substitution should be fairly easy.

Additional Resources/Websites

American Academy of Allergy, Asthma, and Immunology: www.aaaai .org

American College of Allergy, Asthma and Immunology: www.acaai .org

Asthma and Allergy Foundation of America: www.aafa.org

The Food Allergy and Anaphylaxis Network: www.foodallergy.org

Lactose Restricted Diet

Use

The Lactose Restricted Diet is used for people who cannot digest lactose, the carbohydrate found in milk. Lactose intolerance results from diminished production of lactase enzyme in the small intestine. The degree of sensitivity will vary from person to person; consequently the diet should be individualized.

Adequacy

The diet will provide quantities of nutrients recommended by the National Academy of Sciences for adults except for calcium, riboflavin, and vitamin D. Supplementary sources of calcium, riboflavin, and vitamin D may be advisable.

Diet Principles

1. The diet limits lactose-containing foods according to individual tolerance. Foods with small amounts of lactose are often tolerated when eaten in small portions or as part of a meal. Fermented dairy products like yogurt and aged cheeses are often tolerated.
2. Read all labels carefully to identify foods containing lactose. Look for the words *lactose, milk, non-fat dry milk, milk solids, skim milk, whey,* or *curds.* Other prepared foods that may contain lactose include commercial breads and baked goods, processed breakfast cereals, instant potatoes, soup and breakfast drink mixes, margarine, lunchmeats (other than kosher), salad dressings, candies and snacks, mixes for pancakes, biscuits, and cookies.
3. Many prescriptions and over-the-counter medications contain lactose. Check labels or consult with a pharmacist. Commercially

available lactase enzyme (Lactaid, Dairy Ease) may be taken with food, beverages, and some medications as needed.

4. Calcium may be supplemented to provide 1,000–1,500 mg/day as needed. Refer to Appendix 8 for non-dairy food sources of calcium.

FOOD FOR THE DAY

	Allowed	Include as Tolerated
Milk 2–3 cups	Soy milk, lactose-free dairy substitutes; milk treated with lactase enzyme, e.g., Lactaid	Milk and milk products; buttermilk, acidophilus milk, yogurt, cocoa mixes
Meat and Beans 2–3 servings	All fresh meat, poultry, fish, shellfish; eggs; peanut butter, dried beans, lentils; nuts, seeds, tofu, aged cheeses, kosher prepared meat products	Meat or meat substitute prepared with milk; cold cuts, wieners, or other meat with added lactose; powdered eggs, other block cheeses, cottage cheese
Fruits 1–2 ½ cups	All fruits and fruit juices	Fruit drinks containing lactose
Vegetables 1–4 cups (including potatoes)	All vegetables and vegetable juices	Any vegetable prepared with milk or cheese sauce; instant potatoes
Grains 3–10 servings	Crackers, rusk, Italian, French, or Jewish rye bread; cereals except those listed to avoid; rice, pasta, hominy, oats, barley, wheat, cornmeal, tortillas, rice and popcorn cakes	Any bread, cereal, or grain prepared with milk or milk products; instant cereals; dry cereals containing lactose or milk
Oils/Fat	Milk-free margarine (kosher margarines do not contain milk); some nondairy cream substitutes; mayonnaise, vegetable oils, shortening, lard, bacon, salad dressings made without milk or cheese olives; gravy made without milk	Butter, margarine containing milk; salad dressings containing milk; mayonnaise-type salad dressings; sour cream, cream cheese, cream
Sweets/Desserts	Desserts made without milk; fruit ices, popsicles, gelatin; angel food cake, fruit rollups, sugar, corn syrup, maple syrup, honey, jam, jelly; marshmallows; hard candies, gum drops, jelly beans; fruit pie fillings	Any dessert, pudding or mix containing lactose; sherbet, ice cream, frozen yogurt; milk chocolate, caramels, cream or chocolate candies; artificial sweeteners containing lactose

(continued)

FOOD FOR THE DAY *(continued)*

	Allowed	Include as Tolerated
Fluids/Soup	Broth-based soups; soups made with water, soy milk or lactaid, treated milk; plain coffee, tea; soft drinks; beer, wine, distilled spirits; cocoa powder	Cream soups, commercial soups containing milk or lactose; drink mixes containing milk or lactose; Ovaltine; chocolate drink mixes; Instant Breakfast
Others	Popcorn, pretzels, plain potato and corn chips; condiments without added milk	Cheese flavored crackers, cheese curls

Source: The University of Iowa Hospitals & Clinics, Food & Nutrition Services Lactose Restricted Diet, 2002

SUGGESTED MENU PLAN FOR LACTOSE RESTRICTED DIET

 The menu plan for the General Diet should be used. Milk substitutes and milk-free foods as suggested above should be used where appropriate.

Additional Resources/Websites

American Gastroenterology Association: www.gastro.org/lactose

Burlant, A. 1996. *Secrets of Lactose-Free Cooking*. New Hyde Park, NY: Avery Publishing Group.

Dobler, M. L. 1991. rev. 1997. *Lactose Intolerance*. Chicago, IL: ADA.

Inman-Felton, A.E. 1998. Overview of Lactose Maldigestion. *J Am Diet Assoc*. Chicago, IL:ADA.

Martens, R. A. 1987. *The Milk Sugar Dilemma*, 2nd ed. Lansing, MI: Medi-Ed Press.

Swagerty Jr, D.L, et al. 2002. Lactose Intolerance *American Family Physician*. 65:9.

Zukin, J. 1998. *Dairy-Free Cookbook*, 2nd ed. Rocklin, CA: Prima Publishing and Communications.

Gluten Restricted Diet

Use

The Gluten Restricted Diet is used for people with celiac disease, gluten-induced enteropathy, or dermatitis herpetiformis.

Adequacy

The suggested food plan includes foods in amounts that will provide the quantities of nutrients recommended by the National Academy of Sciences for adults. Patients may have malabsorption problems, therefore calorie, protein, vitamin, and mineral intake should be monitored with optimal energy and nutrient intake provided.

Diet Principles

1. This diet restricts gluten by avoiding foods, beverages, and medications containing wheat, rye, oats, and barley.
2. Grains and starches that may be used include corn, rice, potato, soy, tapioca, bean, sorghum, amaranth, buckwheat, quinoa, teff, millet, Montina, and nut flours.
3. It is important to carefully read ingredient labels on all prepared foods to determine possible gluten content. Ingredients such as modified food starch, hydrolyzed or texturized vegetable proteins, soy sauce or soy sauce solids, and malt or malt flavoring may indicate gluten content from an unacceptable source.
4. Care to avoid cross contamination in food preparation is essential.
5. A registered dietitian familiar with the gluten restrictions can assist in diet planning and education to assure nutritional adequacy.

FOOD FOR THE DAY

	Allowed	Foods to Avoid
Milk 2–3 cups	All regular milk or milk treated with lactase enzyme, e.g. Lactaid; yogurt; cream, sour cream, whipping cream	Commercial chocolate and malted milk drinks
Meat and Beans 2–3 servings	All fresh meat, poultry, shellfish, fish; dried beans, peas, lentils; eggs, nuts, peanut butter; tofu; some processed meats, fish, or poultry; block or hard cheeses, cottage cheese	Creamed or breaded meat, fish, poultry unless made with allowed flours; commercial products containing restricted grains; some canned meat products; cold cuts unless all meat; cheese spreads; basted or injected meats and poultry; veined cheese e.g. blue, stilton
Fruits 1–2½ cups	All fruits and fruit juices	Any fruit containing wheat flour used as a thickener
Vegetables 1–4 cups (including potatoes)	All vegetables and vegetable juices; potatoes, sweet potatoes, yams; hominy; some canned baked beans	Creamed or breaded vegetables; some canned baked beans

(continued)

FOOD FOR THE DAY *(continued)*

	Allowed	Foods to Avoid
Grains 3–10 servings	Rice, wild rice; gluten-free breads, cereals, quick breads; gluten-free pasta, noodles; rice flour, potato flour, tapioca starch, quinoa, teff, amaranth, buckwheat, millet, popcorn	Any made with wheat, rye, oats, barley; triticale, spelt, wheat germ, wheat starch, graham, durum, semolina, couscous, malt, kaska, bulgur kamut
Oils/Fat	Margarine, butter, vegetable oils; some salad dressings; some mayonnaise	Any salad dressings or mayonnaise containing restricted grains
Sweets/Desserts	Cakes, cookies, pastries made with gluten-free grains; some pudding mixes; sorbet and fruit ices; premium ice cream; gelatin; some candy; sugar, corn syrup, maple syrup, jam, jelly; marshmallows; some candy and gum; some pie filling	Cakes, cookies, pastries made with restricted grains, ice cream cones; some pudding mixes; ice cream containing bakery goods; some pie fillings
Fluids/Soup	Homemade broths and soups made with allowed ingredients; plain coffee, tea; some soymilk and rice milk; some soft drinks; wine rum, tequila, vodka made from potatoes	Cereal beverages; flavored instant coffees; Postum; Ovaltine; ale, beer, gin, whiskey, vodka, malt liquor; soups thickened or made with restricted grains
Others	Pure herbs and spices; salt, pepper; popcorn; corn tortillas; some plain potato and corn chips; yeast, baking powder, baking soda; some condiments	Some condiments; some herb or spice mixtures

Source: The University of Iowa Hospital & Clinics, Food & Nutrition Services, Gluten-Free Diet, 2002.

SUGGESTED MENU PLAN FOR GLUTEN RESTRICTED DIET

(Select from foods described)

Breakfast

Fruit or fruit juice

Egg

Rice or corn cereal

Gluten-free bread or rusk

Margarine

Milk

Coffee or tea

Lunch or Dinner

Meat or meat substitute

Potato, rice, corn, or gluten-free pasta

Vegetable or salad

Rice cake or gluten-free bread or roll

Margarine or gluten-free salad dressing

Fruit, gluten-free cookies, sherbet, or gluten-free ice cream

Milk

Coffee or tea

Snacks

Any meat or cheese

Rice or corn crackers

Popped corn

Fruits

Vegetables

Milk or gluten-free yogurt

Additional Resources

Murray, J. A. 1999. The Widening Spectrum of Celiac Disease. *Am J Clin Nutr*. 69:354–365.

Thompson, T., Dobler, M.L. 2003. *Celiac Disease Nutrition Guide*. Chicago, IL: ADA.

University of Iowa Hospitals and Clinics. Gluten-free Shopping List. Food and Nutrition Services. Phone: 319-356-3466.

Websites

Celiac.com (internet support site): www.celiac.com

Celiac Sprue Association/United States of America: www.csaceliacs .org

Gluten Intolerance Group: www.gluten.net

Tri-County Celiac Sprue Support Group (source of annually updated shopping list): www.tccsg.com

Phenylalanine Restricted Diet

Use

The phenylalanine restricted diet is used for people who lack the enzyme necessary to convert phenylalanine to tyrosine, causing a disorder called phenylketonuria or PKU. High amounts of phenylalanine are toxic to the brain and can cause mental retardation. Prior to new-born screening (most states started to screen in the 1960s), individuals with PKU were not identified until the brain damage had occurred. Even though a phenylalanine restricted diet will not reverse the mental retardation that may have occurred, it may reduce some of the behavior problems these individuals may have. When newborn screening began, infants were placed on the diet at diagnosis and kept on the diet until 5–8 years of age when it was thought safe to go off the diet because the most rapid time of brain development was over. As more individuals have been off the diet for longer periods of time, it is apparent that high amounts of phenylalanine continue to be a brain toxin and can cause varying degrees of brain damage. Currently, individuals begin the diet at diagnosis and the recommendation is to continue the diet for life so brain damage does not occur.

Adequacy

Depending on the type of the special metabolic formula used, the suggested food plan may provide the quantities of nutrients recommended by the National Academy of Sciences or may need to be supplemented with a multivitamin and calcium supplement.

Diet Principles

1. The diet eliminates all foods containing natural protein such as meat, fish, poultry, milk, yogurt, cheese, eggs, nuts, seeds, legumes, peanut butter.
2. Foods containing aspartame are also eliminated because one of the byproducts of aspartame is phenylalanine. Sucralose and saccharin are allowed.
3. Adequate protein intake is achieved with the use of a metabolic formula that has the phenylalanine removed while the rest of the amino acids remain. Most of the metabolic formulas also provide fat, carbohydrate, vitamins, and minerals.
4. A prescribed amount of phenylalanine is allowed from natural food sources like fruits, vegetables, and grain products.
5. Low protein foods such as pastas, breads, and other baked goods are available to provide calories and variety to the diet without too much phenylalanine.
6. A registered dietitian familiar with the PKU diet should assist in diet planning and teaching to assure nutritional adequacy.

FOOD FOR THE DAY

	Allowed	Foods to Avoid
Milk	Special metabolic formula in the amount prescribed by registered dietitian	All regular milk, yogurt, cheese
Meat and Beans	None	All meat, poultry, fish, eggs, dried beans or peas or peanut butter
Fruits 1-2 ½ cups	Fresh, frozen, canned, dried, fruit juices	None
Vegetables 1–4 cups	All fresh, frozen, canned	Baked beans and other legumes
Grains Amount specified by registered dietitian	All that will fit within protein allotment. May need to use low protein grains	None
Oils/Fat	All are allowed	None
Sweets/Desserts	All that will fit into the protein allotment which may include gelatin, sorbets, fruit ices	Those too high in protein
Fluids	Water and other fluids, such as coffee, tea, fruit or vegetable juice, lemonade, regular soda	Beverages containing aspartame

SUGGESTED MENU PLAN FOR PHENYLALANINE RESTRICTED DIET

(Select from foods described)

Breakfast

Special metabolic formula

Fruit or fruit juice

Cereal

Toast*

Margarine/jelly

Coffee or tea

Lunch or Dinner

Special metabolic formula

Potato, rice, pasta*

Vegetable

Fruit

Cake or cookies*, sorbets, sherbets, gelatin

Coffee or tea

Snacks

Fruit

Hunt's lemon pudding

(continued)

Snacks *(continued)*

Candy with no protein

Low protein baked items

Fruit drinks

Fruit snacks

Popsicles

*Regular or low protein depending on protein allotment

Additional Resources/Websites

Acosta, P, Yannicelli, S. 2001. *The Ross Metabolic Formula System Nutrition Support Protocols*. Columbus, OH: Ross Products Division.

National PKU News: www.pkunews.org

Phenylketonuria: Screening and Management. NIH Consensus Statement Online 2000 October 16–18; 17(3): 1–27.

Schuett, V. 2002. *Low Protein Food List for PKU*. Distributed by SHS North America, Gaithersburg, MD.

Guidelines for Peptic Ulcer, GERD, and Hiatal Hernia

Peptic Ulcer

There is no evidence that a bland diet plays a significant role in the treatment of gastrointestinal disorders. Historically, such a diet was recommended in the treatment of peptic ulcer disease, hiatal hernia, and gastroesophageal reflux disease (GERD). It is now known that most stomach ulcers are caused either by infection with a bacterium called *Helicobacter pylori* (*H.pylori*) or by use of pain medications such as aspirin, ibuprofen, and other non-steroidal anti-inflammatory drugs (NSAID). Most *H.pylori*-related ulcers can be cured with antibiotics. NSAID-induced ulcers can be cured with time, stomach protective medications, antacids, and avoidance of NSAIDs.

No evidence supports the use of a traditional bland diet to decrease gastric acid secretion or increase the rate of healing. For this reason, the diet should be primarily one that is liberal and individualized since patients differ as to specific food intolerances. There are a few foods that can stimulate gastric secretion and possibly irritate the stomach. It is a very limited list and should be based on patient tolerance along with lifestyle changes for the treatment of peptic ulcers. The following recommendations are made:

1. Avoid alcohol, cigarette smoking, salicylates (aspirin), and other non-steroidal anti-inflammatory drug (NSAID) agents.

2. Avoid frequent meals and or bedtime snacks to prevent increased acid secretion.
3. Foods and seasonings that stimulate gastric acid secretion such as caffeine, black pepper, garlic, cloves, and chili powder should be limited.

Gastroesophageal Reflux Disease (GERD) and Hiatal Hernia

Hiatal hernia occurs when a portion of the stomach bulges up into the esophagus. This causes reflux of stomach contents, resulting in heartburn and a bitter or sour taste in the back of the throat. When this happens frequently it is called Gastroesophageal Reflux Disease or GERD. If left untreated, GERD can cause damage to the lining of the esophagus.

Lifestyle modifications, medications, and diet can manage the symptoms of this disease. The following recommendations are made:

1. Avoid foods and beverages that contribute to indigestion: chocolate, coffee, and other highly caffeinated beverages; peppermint; high fat or spicy foods; tomato products; and alcoholic beverages. Some sources also suggest limiting citrus fruits.
2. Stop smoking to reduce the effect of tobacco on stomach acid production and relaxation of the esophageal muscles. Tobacco also inhibits saliva, which is the body's major buffer.
3. Avoid drinking alcohol.
4. Reduce weight if obese.
5. Avoid eating 2–3 hours before sleep.
6. Raise the head of the bed by 6 inches.

SUGGESTED MENU PLAN FOR PEPTIC ULCER, GERD, HIATAL HERNIA

(Select from foods described)

Breakfast

Fruit or juice*

Cereal with milk and/or egg

Toast with margarine or butter

Beverage-decaffeinated

Midmorning

Milk

Cookie or cracker

Lunch or Supper

Soup or juice*, as desired

(continued)

Lunch or Supper *(continued)*

Meat or meat substitute

Vegetable, cooked

Bread with margarine or butter

Light dessert, such as pudding or sherbet

Milk

Midafternoon

Yogurt

Beverage

Dinner

Meat or meat substitute

Potato, pasta, or grain

Vegetable, cooked

Bread with margarine or butter

Fruit*

Milk

*If tolerated

References/Websites

American College of Gastroenterology: www.acg.gi.org/patients

American Dietetic Association position paper: bland diets. 1971. *J Am Diet Assoc.* 59(3):244–5.

The Cleveland Clinic Digestive Disease Center: www.clevelandclinic .org/digestivedisease

Mayo Clinic: www.mayoclinic.com/health/pepticulcer/DS00242

National Institute of diabetes and digestive disorders: www.digestive .niddk.nih.gov

Study Guide Questions

A. List at least three uses for the High Nutrient Diet.

B. The suggested food plan for the High Nutrient Diet includes foods in amounts that will provide _____, _____, _____, and _____ in amounts greater than recommended by the National Academy of Sciences for adults.

C. List at least three foods that are high in vitamin C. Refer to the vitamin C foods listed in Chapter 1 under the Fruit Group category.

D. List at least three foods that are high in zinc. Refer to "Zinc Content of Selected Foods" in Appendix 9.

E. List at least three ways in which calories, protein, and vitamins can be added without increasing portion size.

F. Modify the general menu planned in Chapter 2 to increase protein and calorie content with little change in portion size.

G. Describe in detail at least three diet principles related to the Finger Food Modification Diet.

H. List four types of vegetarian diets.

I. When planning vegetarian diets, why should the following be given special consideration?

- Protein
- Calcium
- Iron
- Vitamin B-12

J. Define the following:

- Food allergy
- Food intolerance

K. List at least four common food allergies.

L. Lactose intolerance results from what?

M. List at least three prepared foods that may contain lactose.

N. List at least three grains and starches that may be used for Gluten Restricted Diets.

O. When reading food labels, what ingredients listed would indicate possible gluten content? (Hint: modified food starch)

P. Describe in detail at least three diet principles associated with the Phenylalanine Restricted Diet.

Q. List at least three lifestyle changes that may be helpful for patients with peptic ulcers or GERD.

CHAPTER 12

Dining Assistance/
Special Needs

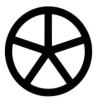

Feeding Guidelines for Individuals with Dementia

Individuals with dementia are at risk for weight loss and poor nutritional intake. Caregivers need to be flexible with their feeding strategies and allow as much time as needed at the mealtime. Encourage the individual to do as much for themselves as possible, but provide adequate assistance and support for them to be successful. Feeding assistance should be provided as needed; watch for body cues and offer sensitivity to their feelings. Feeding approaches need to be tailored to the individual. Allow for family involvement at mealtimes; they can also offer vital input into food preferences and possible feeding strategies that may work with an individual.

The following is a non-exclusive list of feeding guidelines to consider at mealtimes to promote safe oral intake and a positive feeding environment:

1. Maintain an upright position. Have the client sit up in a chair with feet supported on the floor, a foot rest, or a foot stool. If the client must be fed in bed or a Geri chair, raise the head of the bed or use pillows. Pillows under the legs and a 90-degree bend at the hips are often helpful. Clients should remain upright for at least 20 minutes after meals to prevent reflux.
2. Reduce the risk of aspiration by avoiding tilting the head. Caregivers should sit at eye level to promote a chin tuck swallow.
3. Avoid the use of syringes. Syringe feeding rapidly forces liquified food to the back of the throat and increases the risk of aspiration. In addition, the inherent dignity of the individual is greatly reduced.
4. Focus on the resident. Avoid inappropriate conversation and distractions.

5. Check for pocketing of food during and after the meal.

6. Offer small bites and sips, alternate liquids and solids to promote a safe swallow. Be sure food has been completely swallowed before offering a beverage.

7. Provide foods that stimulate appetite by their appearance, smell, and taste. Identify the food as you give it. Make positive remarks, such as "Doesn't this look good?!" or "That smells good!"

8. Try alternating warm and cold foods. Enhance the flavor of food with condiments and seasonings for sensory stimulation and to improve food palatability.

9. Allow plenty of time to eat. If a meal cannot be eaten in 30 to 45 minutes, consider serving smaller, more frequent meals. Longer mealtimes may tire the client and put him/her at increased risk for swallowing problems.

10. Observe and report swallowing complications, i.e., coughing, throat clearing, abnormal rate of eating, pocketing food or spilling food/liquids from the mouth. Foods with combination textures—such as chunky soups or dry cereal with milk—and foods that are crumbly and fall apart easily—such as corn, peas, and rice—are the most difficult to swallow safely.

11. Do not use straws unless approved by the speech or occupational therapist. For some clients, the use of a straw forcefully propels the liquid to the back of the throat before the normal swallow reflex is triggered.

12. Feeding a client the first few bites of food may "prime" self-feeding behavior, after which you can hand the spoon to the client. Consider hand over hand technique.

13. Try offering one food item and beverage at a time; the client may benefit from reduction in decision making.

14. Promote a consistent seating arrangement to provide familiarity and lessen anxiety. Eating with a group at a table can keep the client on task.

Additional Resource

Hellen CR. 1998. *Alzheimer's Disease Activity-Focused Care*, 2nd edition. Woburn, MA: Butterworth-Heinemann.

Nutrition for Individuals with Developmental Disabilities

Developmental disabilities include varied diagnoses, including congenital anomalies, neuromuscular dysfunction, genetic or metabolic syndromes, chronic health conditions, and behavioral disorders. Baer and other have developed a table for types of nutrition problems often seen with individual disorders. (11)

■ INDIVIDUALIZATION

Persons with the same diagnosis may have different dietary needs. Standard nutrition guidelines (age, gender specific) can be applied and individualized to meet nutritional needs.

■ ENERGY REQUIREMENTS

Calorie requirements commonly are lower than the general population. High muscle tone and abnormal muscle movements may increase calorie needs. Body height (calories per centimeter) is often used to determine energy requirements instead of weight (calories per kilogram). General guidelines for normal growth and weight maintenance often range from 12 to 15 calories per centimeter of body height, and 10 calories or less per centimeter of body height is required to promote weight loss. Documenting and monitoring weight status on a regular basis is important to determine individual calorie needs. Some specialized growth charts for children with disabilities are available to use in assessing growth and weight gain. Syndrome associations usually provide access to growth charts, i.e. National Down Syndrome Society.

■ MACRONUTRIENT COMPOSITION

In most cases carbohydrate, protein, and fat distribution does not differ from recommendations made for the general population. In specific metabolic disorders, special low protein and/or low fat diets are required.

■ VITAMINS/MINERALS

Diagnosis-specific conditions may require prescribed vitamin and/or mineral supplementation, i.e., cystic fibrosis, congenital heart disorders and rheumatoid arthritis. For individuals on long-term medications (seizure drugs) or for those that have eliminated entire food groups (allergies, autism), supplementation of vitamins/minerals may be indicated.

◼ FEEDING PROBLEMS

Feeding problems are common for individuals with neuromuscular conditions. Dysphagia (oral motor dysfunction), nasopharyngeal reflux, constipation, esophageal dysmotility, gastroesophageal reflux, and delayed gastric emptying are common causes of feeding problems. An individual with abnormal muscle movement may never progress to normal food textures, but therapy for delayed feeding skills (normal muscle movement) may help improve dietary intake. Significant food refusals may be an indicator of various problems (sensory, pain, etc.) and should be evaluated by an interdisciplinary feeding team.

◼ BEHAVIORAL FEEDING CONCERNS

Individuals who are not verbal may use behavior as communication. Medical causes of pain should be resolved (gastroesphogeal reflux) prior to psychological intervention. Behavior problems can also occur when caregiver expectations for self-feeding or diet textures are higher than cognitive and motor abilities of the individual allow.

◼ ENTERAL FEEDINGS

Dependency upon formula or high calorie liquid supplements— either in combination with oral food intake or as the primary source of nutrition—is common. With low calorie needs, standard formulas may require protein or micronutrient supplementation. Additional water may be necessary to maintain adequate fluid volume. Fiber-containing formulas promote good bowel management in individuals with neuromuscular conditions.

◼ ALTERNATIVE NUTRITION

Families and/or individuals with disabilities and chronic health conditions are subject to nutrition misinformation and unsubstantiated health claims. Nutrition assessment should include complete documentation and evaluation of special dietary regimens and supplements along with possible drug/nutrient interactions.

◼ PHYSICAL ACTIVITY

People with disabilities are less likely to engage in regular physical activity but have similar health needs for activity. Non-ambulatory conditions increase risk of obesity, pressure sores, osteoporosis, and cardiovascular and respiratory problems. Daily physical activity is recommended; strategies can be developed to fit individual abilities.

Additional Resources/Websites

Ekvall SW, ed. 1993. *Pediatric Nutrition in Chronic Diseases and Developmental Disorders*. New York, NY: Oxford University Press.

Iowa's University Center for Excellence on Disabilities: www.healthcare.uiowa.edu/cdd/multiple/iuce/ucedd.asp

Iowa's Title V Program for CSHCN: www.uihealthcare.com/depts/state/chsc/index.html

Lucas BL, Feucht SA, Grieger LE, ed. 2004. *Children with Special Health Care Needs Nutrition Care Handbook*. Chicago, IL: ADA.

National Center for Physical Activity and Disability: www.ncpad.org/index.php

The National Down Syndrome Society: www.ndss.org/content.cfm

Position of the American Dietetic Association: nutrition services for children with special health needs. 1995. *J Am Diet Assoc*. 95:809–817.

The Surgeon General's Call to Action to Improve the Health and Wellness of Persons with Disabilities: www.surgeongeneral.gov/library/disabilities/

Washington State Department of Health. 2001. *Nutrition Interventions for Children with Special Health Care Needs*. March: Publication No. 961–158.

Study Guide Questions

A. Describe in detail six guidelines for feeding individuals with dementia.

B. If your facility has a dining room for individuals with dementia, observe two meals. Compare your findings with the guidelines presented. What practices are being implemented in your facility? Discuss your findings with the dietitian or food service manager and make recommendations for change.

C. If your facility has a dining room for patients with developmental disabilities, observe two meals. Discuss your findings with the dietitian or food service manager. What individual dietary modifications are being used? What is the rationale for these modifications? How are feeding and behavioral problems being addressed?

APPENDIXES

1.

DIETARY REFERENCE INTAKES (DRIs): RECOMMENDED INTAKES FOR INDIVIDUALS, VITAMINS

Food and Nutrition Board, Institute of Medicine, National Academies

Life Stage Group	Vit A (μg/d)[a]	Vit C (mg/d)	Vit D (μg/d)[b,c]	Vit E (mg/d)[d]	Vit K (μg/d)	Thiamin (mg/d)	Riboflavin (mg/d)	Niacin (mg/d)[e]	Vit B$_6$ (mg/d)	Folate (μg/d)[f]	Vit B$_{12}$ (μg/d)	Pantothenic Acid (mg/d)	Biotin (μg/d)	Choline[g] (mg/d)
Infants														
0–6 mo	400*	40*	5*	4*	2.0*	0.2*	0.3*	2*	0.1*	65*	0.4*	1.7*	5*	125*
7–12 mo	500*	50*	5*	5*	2.5*	0.3*	0.4*	4*	0.3*	80*	0.5*	1.8*	6*	150*
Children														
1–3 y	300	15	5*	6	30*	0.5	0.5	6	0.5	150	0.9	2*	8*	200*
4–8 y	400	25	5*	7	55*	0.6	0.6	8	0.6	200	1.2	3*	12*	250*
Males														
9–13 y	600	45	5*	11	60*	0.9	0.9	12	1.0	300	1.8	4*	20*	375*
14–18 y	900	75	5*	15	75*	1.2	1.3	16	1.3	400	2.4	5*	25*	550*
19–30 y	900	90	5*	15	120*	1.2	1.3	16	1.3	400	2.4	5*	30*	550*
31–50 y	900	90	5*	15	120*	1.2	1.3	16	1.3	400	2.4	5*	30*	550*
51–70 y	900	90	10*	15	120*	1.2	1.3	16	1.7	400	2.4[h]	5*	30*	550*
>70 y	900	90	15*	15	120*	1.2	1.3	16	1.7	400	2.4[h]	5*	30*	550*
Females														
9–13 y	600	45	5*	11	60*	0.9	0.9	12	1.0	300	1.8	4*	20*	375*
14–18 y	700	65	5*	15	75*	1.0	1.0	14	1.2	400[i]	2.4	5*	25*	400*
19–30 y	700	75	5*	15	90*	1.1	1.1	14	1.3	400[i]	2.4	5*	30*	425*
31–50 y	700	75	5*	15	90*	1.1	1.1	14	1.3	400[i]	2.4	5*	30*	425*
51–70 y	700	75	10*	15	90*	1.1	1.1	14	1.5	400	2.4[h]	5*	30*	425*
>70 y	700	75	15*	15	90*	1.1	1.1	14	1.5	400	2.4[h]	5*	30*	425*
Pregnancy														
14-18 y	750	80	5*	15	75*	1.4	1.4	18	1.9	600[j]	2.6	6*	30*	450*
19-30 y	770	85	5*	15	90*	1.4	1.4	18	1.9	600[j]	2.6	6*	30*	450*
31-50 y	770	85	5*	15	90*	1.4	1.4	18	1.9	600[j]	2.6	6*	30*	450*
Lactation														
14-18 y	1,200	115	5*	19	75*	1.4	1.6	17	2.0	500	2.8	7*	35*	550*
19-30 y	1,300	120	5*	19	90*	1.4	1.6	17	2.0	500	2.8	7*	35*	550*
31-50 y	1,300	120	5*	19	90*	1.4	1.6	17	2.0	500	2.8	7*	35*	550*

DIETARY REFERENCE INTAKES (DRIs): RECOMMENDED INTAKES FOR INDIVIDUALS, VITAMINS

NOTE: This table (taken from the DRI reports, see www.nap.edu) presents Recommended Dietary Allowances (RDAs) in **bold type** and Adequate Intakes (AIs) in ordinary type followed by an asterisk (*). RDAs and AIs may both be used as goals for individual intake. RDAs are set to meet the needs of almost all (97 to 98 percent) individuals in a group. For healthy breastfed infants, the AI is the mean intake. The AI for other life stage and gender groups is believed to cover needs of all individuals in the group, but lack of data or uncertainty in the data prevent being able to specify with confidence the percentage of individuals covered by this intake.

a As retinol activity equivalents (RAEs). 1 RAE = 1 μg retinol, 12 μg β-carotene, 24 μg a-carotene, or 24 μg β-cryptoxanthin. The RAE for dietary provitamin A carotenoids is twofold greater than retinol equivalents (RE), whereas the RAE for preformed vitamin A is the same as RE.

b cholecalciferol. 1 μg cholecalciferol = 40 IU vitamin D.

c In the absence of adequate exposure to sunlight.

d As a-tocopherol. a-Tocopherol includes RRR-a-tocopherol, the only form of a-tocopherol that occurs naturally in foods, and the 2R-stereoisomeric forms of a-tocopherol (RRR-, RSR-, RRS-, and RSS-a-tocopherol) that occur in fortified foods and supplements. It does not include the 2S-stereoisomeric forms of a-tocopherol (SRR-, SSR-, SRS-, and SSS-a-tocopherol), also found in fortified foods and supplements.

e As niacin equivalents (NE). 1 mg of niacin = 60 mg of tryptophan; 0–6 months = preformed niacin (not NE).

f As dietary folate equivalents (DFE). 1 DFE = 1 μg food folate = 0.6 μg of folic acid from fortified food or as a supplement consumed with food = 0.5 μg of a supplement taken on an empty stomach.

g Although AIs have been set for choline, there are few data to assess whether a dietary supply of choline is needed at all stages of the life cycle, and it may be that the choline requirement can be met by endogenous synthesis at some of these stages.

h Because 10 to 30 percent of older people may malabsorb food-bound B_{12}, it is advisable for those older than 50 years to meet their RDA mainly by consuming foods fortified with B_{12} or a supplement containing B_{12}.

i In view of evidence linking folate intake with neural tube defects in the fetus, it is recommended that all women capable of becoming pregnant consume 400 μg from supplements or fortified foods in addition to intake of food folate from a varied diet.

j It is assumed that women will continue consuming 400 μg from supplements or fortified food until their pregnancy is confirmed and they enter prenatal care, which ordinarily occurs after the end of the periconceptional period—the critical time for formation of the neural tube.

2.

DIETARY REFERENCE INTAKES (DRIs): TOLERABLE UPPER INTAKE LEVELS (UL^a), VITAMINS

Food and Nutrition Board, Institute of Medicine, National Academies

Life Stage Group	Vit A (µg/d)^b	Vit C (mg/d)	Vit D (mg/d)	Vit E (mg/d)^{c,d}	Vit K	Thiamin	Ribo-flavin	Niacin (mg/d)^d	Vitamin B$_6$ (mg/d)	Folate (µg/d)^d	Vit B$_{12}$	Panto-thenic Acid	Biotin	Choline (g/d)	Carote-noids^e
Infants															
0–6 mo	600	ND^f	25	ND	ND	ND	ND	ND	ND	ND	ND	ND	ND	ND	ND
7–12 mo	600	ND	25	ND	ND	ND	ND	ND	ND	ND	ND	ND	ND	ND	ND
Children																
1–3 y	600	400	50	200	ND	ND	ND	10	30	300	ND	ND	ND	1.0	ND
4–8 y	900	650	50	300	ND	ND	ND	15	40	400	ND	ND	ND	1.0	ND
Males, Females																
9–13 y	1,700	1,200	50	600	ND	ND	ND	20	60	600	ND	ND	ND	2.0	ND
14–18 y	2,800	1,800	50	800	ND	ND	ND	30	80	800	ND	ND	ND	3.0	ND
19–70 y	3,000	2,000	50	1,000	ND	ND	ND	35	100	1,000	ND	ND	ND	3.5	ND
> 70 y	3,000	2,000	50	1,000	ND	ND	ND	35	100	1,000	ND	ND	ND	3.5	ND
Pregnancy																
14–18 y	2,800	1,800	50	800	ND	ND	ND	30	80	800	ND	ND	ND	3.0	ND
19–50 y	3,000	2,000	50	1,000	ND	ND	ND	35	100	1,000	ND	ND	ND	3.5	ND
Lactation																
14–18 y	2,800	1,800	50	800	ND	ND	ND	30	80	800	ND	ND	ND	3.0	ND
19–50 y	3,000	2,000	50	1,000	ND	ND	ND	35	100	1,000	ND	ND	ND	3.5	ND

^{a} UL = The maximum level of daily nutrient intake that is likely to pose no risk of adverse effects. Unless otherwise specified, the UL represents total intake from food, water, and supplements. Due to lack of suitable data, ULs could not be established for vitamin K, thiamin, riboflavin, vitamin B$_{12}$, pantothenic acid, biotin, or carotenoids. In the absence of ULs, extra caution may be warranted in consuming levels above recommended intakes.

^{b} As preformed vitamin A only.

^{c} As a-tocopherol; applies to any form of supplemental a-tocopherol.

^{d} The ULs for vitamin E, niacin, and folate apply to synthetic forms obtained from supplements, fortified foods, or a combination of the two.

^{e} β-Carotene supplements are advised only to serve as a provitamin A source for individuals at risk of vitamin A deficiency.

^{f} ND = Not determinable due to lack of data of adverse effects in this age group and concern with regard to lack of ability to handle excess amounts. Source of intake should be from food only to prevent high levels of intake.

Copyright 2004 by the National Academy of Sciences. All rights reserved.

3.

DIETARY REFERENCE INTAKES: RECOMMENDED INTAKES FOR INDIVIDUALS, ELEMENTS

Food and Nutrition Board, Institute of Medicine, National Academies

Life Stage Group	Calcium (mg/d)	Chromium (µg/d)	Copper (µg/d)	Fluoride (mg/d)	Iodine (µg/d)	Iron (mg/d)	Magnesium (mg/d)	Manganese (mg/d)	Molybdenum (µg/d)	Phosphorus (mg/d)	Selenium (µg/d)	Zinc (mg/d)	Potassium (g/d)	Sodium (g/d)	Chloride (g/d)
Infants															
0–6 mo	210*	0.2*	200*	0.01*	110*	0.27*	30*	0.003*	2*	100*	15*	2*	0.4*	0.12*	0.18*
7–12 mo	270*	5.5*	220*	0.5*	130*	11*	75*	0.6*	3*	275*	20*	3*	0.7*	0.37*	0.57*
Children															
1–3 y	500*	11*	340	0.7*	90	7	80	1.2*	17	460	20	3	3.0*	1.0*	1.5*
4–8 y	800*	15*	440	1*	90	10	130	1.5*	22	500	30	5	3.8*	1.2*	1.9*
Males															
9–13 y	1,300*	25*	700	2*	120	8	240	1.9*	34	1,250	40	8	4.5*	1.5*	2.3*
14–18 y	1,300*	35*	890	3*	150	11	410	2.2*	43	1,250	55	11	4.7*	1.5*	2.3*
19–30 y	1,000*	35*	900	4*	150	8	400	2.3*	45	700	55	11	4.7*	1.5*	2.3*
31–50 y	1,000*	35*	900	4*	150	8	420	2.3*	45	700	55	11	4.7*	1.5*	2.3*
51–70 y	1,200*	30*	900	4*	150	8	420	2.3*	45	700	55	11	4.7*	1.3*	2.0*
> 70 y	1,200*	30*	900	4*	150	8	420	2.3*	45	700	55	11	4.7*	1.2*	1.8*
Females															
9–13 y	1,300*	21*	700	2*	120	8	240	1.6*	34	1,250	40	8	4.5*	1.5*	2.3*
14–18 y	1,300*	24*	890	3*	150	15	360	1.6*	43	1,250	55	9	4.7*	1.5*	2.3*
19–30 y	1,000*	25*	900	3*	150	18	310	1.8*	45	700	55	8	4.7*	1.5*	2.3*
31–50 y	1,000*	25*	900	3*	150	18	320	1.8*	45	700	55	8	4.7*	1.5*	2.3*
51–70 y	1,200*	20*	900	3*	150	8	320	1.8*	45	700	55	8	4.7*	1.3*	2.0*
> 70 y	1,200*	20*	900	3*	150	8	320	1.8*	45	700	55	8	4.7*	1.2*	1.8*
Pregnancy															
14–18 y	1,300*	29*	1,000	3*	220	27	400	2.0*	50	1,250	60	12	4.7*	1.5*	2.3*
19–30 y	1,000*	30*	1,000	3*	220	27	350	2.0*	50	700	60	11	4.7*	1.5*	2.3*
31–50 y	1,000*	30*	1,000	3*	220	27	360	2.0*	50	700	60	11	4.7*	1.5*	2.3*

(continued)

3. *(continued)*

DIETARY REFERENCE INTAKES: RECOMMENDED INTAKES FOR INDIVIDUALS, ELEMENTS

Food and Nutrition Board, Institute of Medicine, National Academies

Life Stage Group	Calcium (mg/d)	Chromium (μg/d)	Copper (μg/d)	Fluoride (mg/d)	Iodine (μg/d)	Iron (mg/d)	Magnesium (mg/d)	Manganese (mg/d)	Molybdenum (μg/d)	Phosphorus (mg/d)	Selenium (μg/d)	Zinc (mg/d)	Potassium (g/d)	Sodium (g/d)	Chloride (g/d)
Lactation															
14-18 y	1,300*	44*	1,300	3*	290	10	360	2.6*	50	1,250	70	13	5.1*	1.5*	2.3*
19–30 y	1,000*	45*	1,300	3*	290	9	310	2.6*	50	700	70	12	5.1*	1.5*	2.3*
31–50 y	1,000*	45*	1,300	3*	290	9	320	2.6*	50	700	70	12	5.1*	1.5*	2.3*

NOTE: This table presents Recommended Dietary Allowances (RDAs) in **bold type** and Adequate Intakes (AIs) in ordinary type followed by an asterisk (*). RDAs and AIs may both be used as goals for individual intake. RDAs are set to meet the needs of almost all (97 to 98 percent) individuals in a group. For healthy breastfed infants, the AI is the mean intake. The AI for other life stage and gender groups is believed to cover needs of all individuals in the group, but lack of data or uncertainty in the data prevent being able to specify with confidence the percentage of individuals covered by this intake.

SOURCES: *Dietary Reference Intakes for Calcium, Phosphorous, Magnesium, Vitamin D, and Fluoride* (1997); *Dietary Reference Intakes for Thiamin, Riboflavin, Niacin, Vitamin B_6, Folate, Vitamin B_{12}, Pantothenic Acid, Biotin, and Choline* (1998); *Dietary Reference Intakes for Vitamin C, Vitamin E, Selenium, and Carotenoids* (2000); *Dietary Reference Intakes for Vitamin A, Vitamin K, Arsenic, Boron, Chromium, Copper, Iodine, Iron, Manganese, Molybdenum, Nickel, Silicon, Vanadium, and Zinc* (2001); and *Dietary Reference Intakes for Water, Potassium, Sodium, Chloride, and Sulfate* (2004). These reports may be accessed via www.nap.edu.

4.

DIETARY REFERENCE INTAKES (DRIs): TOLERABLE UPPER INTAKE LEVELS (UL[a]), ELEMENTS

Food and Nutrition Board, Institute of Medicine, National Academies

Life Stage Group	Arsenic[b] (mg/d)	Boron (mg/d)	Calcium (g/d)	Chromium	Copper (μg/d)	Fluoride (mg/d)	Iodine (μg/d)	Iron (mg/d)	Magnesium (mg/d)[c]	Manganese (mg/d)	Molybdenum (μg/d)	Nickel (mg/d)	Phosphorus (g/d)	Potassium	Selenium (μg/d)	Silicon[d]	Sulfate[f]	Vanadium (mg/d)[e]	Zinc (mg/d)	Sodium (g/d)	Chloride (g/d)
Infants																				
0–6 mo	ND[f]	ND	ND	ND	ND	0.7	ND	40	ND	ND	ND	ND	ND	ND	45	ND	ND	ND	4	ND	ND
7–12 mo	ND	ND	ND	ND	ND	0.9	ND	40	ND	ND	ND	ND	ND	ND	60	ND	ND	ND	5	ND	ND
Children																				
1–3 y	ND	3	2.5	ND	1,000	1.3	200	40	65	2	300	0.2	3	ND	90	ND	ND	ND	7	1.5	2.3
4–8 y	ND	6	2.5	ND	3,000	2.2	300	40	110	3	600	0.3	3	ND	150	ND	ND	ND	12	1.9	2.9
Males, Females																				
9–13 y	ND	11	2.5	ND	5,000	10	600	40	350	6	1,100	0.6	4	ND	280	ND	ND	ND	23	2.2	3.4
14–18 y	ND	17	2.5	ND	8,000	10	900	45	350	9	1,700	1.0	4	ND	400	ND	ND	ND	34	2.3	3.6
19–70 y	ND	20	2.5	ND	10,000	10	1,100	45	350	11	2,000	1.0	4	ND	400	ND	ND	1.8	40	2.3	3.6
> 70 y	ND	20	2.5	ND	10,000	10	1,100	45	350	11	2,000	1.0	3	ND	400	ND	ND	1.8	40	2.3	3.6
Pregnancy																				
14–18 y	ND	17	2.5	ND	8,000	10	900	45	350	9	1,700	1.0	3.5	ND	400	ND	ND	ND	34	2.3	3.6
19–50 y	ND	20	2.5	ND	10,000	10	1,100	45	350	11	2,000	1.0	3.5	ND	400	ND	ND	ND	40	2.3	3.6
Lactation																				
14–18 y	ND	17	2.5	ND	8,000	10	900	45	350	9	1,700	1.0	4	ND	400	ND	ND	ND	34	2.3	3.6
19–50 y	ND	20	2.5	ND	10,000	10	1,100	45	350	11	2,000	1.0	4	ND	400	ND	ND	ND	40	2.3	3.6

(continued)

4.

DIETARY REFERENCE INTAKES (DRIs): TOLERABLE UPPER INTAKE LEVELS (UL[a]), ELEMENTS (continued)

[a] UL = The maximum level of daily nutrient intake that is likely to pose no risk of adverse effects. Unless otherwise specified, the UL represents total intake from food, water, and supplements. Due to lack of suitable data, ULs could not be established for arsenic, chromium, silicon, potassium, and sulfate. In the absence of ULs, extra caution may be warranted in consuming levels above recommended intakes.

[b] Although the UL was not determined for arsenic, there is no justification for adding arsenic to food or supplements.

[c] The ULs for magnesium represent intake from a pharmacological agent only and do not include intake from food and water.

[d] Although silicon has not been shown to cause adverse effects in humans, there is no justification for adding silicon to supplements.

[e] Although vanadium in food has not been shown to cause adverse effects in humans, there is no justification for adding vanadium to food and vanadium supplements should be used with caution. The UL is based on adverse effects in laboratory animals and this data could be used to set a UL for adults but not children and adolescents.

[f] ND = Not determinable due to lack of data of adverse effects in this age group and concern with regard to lack of ability to handle excess amounts. Source of intake should be from food only to prevent high levels of intake.

SOURCES: *Dietary Reference Intakes for Calcium, Phosphorous, Magnesium, Vitamin D, and Fluoride* (1997); *Dietary Reference Intakes for Thiamin, Riboflavin, Niacin, Vitamin B₆, Folate, Vitamin B₁₂, Pantothenic Acid, Biotin, and Choline* (1998); *Dietary Reference Intakes for Vitamin C, Vitamin E, Selenium, and Carotenoids* (2000); *Dietary Reference Intakes for Vitamin A, Vitamin K, Arsenic, Boron, Chromium, Copper, Iodine, Iron, Manganese, Molybdenum, Nickel, Silicon, Vanadium, and Zinc* (2001); and *Dietary Reference Intakes for Water, Potassium, Sodium, Chloride, and Sulfate* (2004). These reports may be accessed via www.nap.edu.

5.

Body Mass Index Table (kg/m²) or (lb/in² X 703)

Body Weight (pounds)

Height (inches) / BMI	Normal						Overweight					Obese										Extreme Obesity														
BMI	19	20	21	22	23	24	25	26	27	28	29	30	31	32	33	34	35	36	37	38	39	40	41	42	43	44	45	46	47	48	49	50	51	52	53	54
58	91	96	100	105	110	115	119	124	129	134	138	143	148	153	158	162	167	172	177	181	186	191	196	201	205	210	215	220	224	229	234	239	244	248	253	258
59	94	99	104	109	114	119	124	128	133	138	143	148	153	158	163	168	173	178	183	188	193	198	203	208	212	217	222	227	232	237	242	247	252	257	262	267
60	97	102	107	112	118	123	128	133	138	143	148	153	158	163	168	174	179	184	189	194	199	204	209	215	220	225	230	235	240	245	250	255	261	266	271	276
61	100	106	111	116	122	127	132	137	143	148	153	158	164	169	174	180	185	190	195	201	206	211	217	222	227	232	238	243	248	254	259	264	269	275	280	285
62	104	109	115	120	126	131	136	142	147	153	158	164	169	175	180	186	191	196	202	207	213	218	224	229	235	240	246	251	256	262	267	273	278	284	289	295
63	107	113	118	124	130	135	141	146	152	158	163	169	175	180	186	191	197	203	208	214	220	225	231	237	242	248	254	259	265	270	276	282	287	293	299	304
64	110	116	122	128	134	140	145	151	157	163	169	174	180	186	192	197	204	209	215	221	227	232	238	244	250	256	262	267	273	279	285	291	296	302	308	314
65	114	120	126	132	138	144	150	156	162	168	174	180	186	192	198	204	210	216	222	228	234	240	246	252	258	264	270	276	282	288	294	300	306	312	318	324
66	118	124	130	136	142	148	155	161	167	173	179	186	192	198	204	210	216	223	229	235	241	247	253	260	266	272	278	284	291	297	303	309	315	322	328	334
67	121	127	134	140	146	153	159	166	172	178	185	191	198	204	211	217	223	230	236	242	249	255	261	268	274	280	287	293	299	306	312	319	325	331	338	344
68	125	131	138	144	151	158	164	171	177	184	190	197	203	210	216	223	230	236	243	249	256	262	269	276	282	289	295	302	308	315	322	328	335	341	348	354
69	128	135	142	149	155	162	169	176	182	189	196	203	209	216	223	230	236	243	250	257	263	270	277	284	291	297	304	311	318	324	331	338	345	351	358	365
70	132	139	146	153	160	167	174	181	188	195	202	209	216	222	229	236	243	250	257	264	271	278	285	292	299	306	313	320	327	334	341	348	355	362	369	376
71	136	143	150	157	165	172	179	186	193	200	208	215	222	229	236	243	250	257	265	272	279	286	293	301	308	315	322	329	336	343	351	358	365	372	379	386
72	140	147	154	162	169	177	184	191	199	206	213	221	228	235	242	250	258	265	272	279	287	294	302	309	316	324	331	338	346	353	361	368	375	383	390	397
73	144	151	159	166	174	182	189	197	204	212	219	227	235	242	250	257	265	272	280	288	295	302	310	318	325	333	340	348	355	363	371	378	386	393	401	408
74	148	155	163	171	179	186	194	202	210	218	225	233	241	249	256	264	272	280	287	295	303	311	319	326	334	342	350	358	365	373	381	389	396	404	412	420
75	152	160	168	176	184	192	200	208	216	224	232	240	248	256	264	272	279	287	295	303	311	319	327	335	343	351	359	367	375	383	391	399	407	415	423	431
76	156	164	172	180	189	197	205	213	221	230	238	246	254	263	271	279	287	295	304	312	320	328	336	344	353	361	369	377	385	394	402	410	418	426	435	443

Source: Adapted from *Clinical Guidelines on the Identification, Evaluation, and Treatment of Overweight and Obesity in Adults: The Evidence Report*. National Heart, Blood and Lung Institute, part of the National Institutes of Health and U.S. Department of Health & Human Services BMI Calculator: http:www.nhlbisupport.com/bmi

6. Classifications for BMI

	BMI (kg/m²)
Underweight	<18.5
Normal	18.5–24.9
Overweight	25–29.9
Obesity (Class 1)	30–34.9
Obesity (Class 2)	35–39.9
Extreme obesity (Class 3)	≥40

Source: National Heart, Lung and Blood Institute (part of the National Institutes of Health &
U.S. Dept of Health and Human Services) and North American Association for the Study of
Obesity. Oct 2000. *The Practical Guide: Identification, Evaluation, and Treatment of Overweight and
Obesity in Adults.*

7. Vitamin A Content of Selected Foods

Food Sources of Vitamin A ranked by micrograms Retinol Activity
Equivalents (RAE) of vitamin A per standard amount. The Recommended Dietary Allowance for children 9–13 years of age is 600 μg; females 14 years and older is 700 μg; males 14 years and older is 900 μg.

Food source	Retinol Equivalents (RAE)
Organ meats (liver, giblets), cooked, 1 oz.	477–3,042
Sweet potato, baked in skin, medium	1,403
Braunschweiger, 1 slice	1,197
Pumpkin, canned, ½ cup	953
Carrots, raw, 1 cup	925
Carrots, raw, cooked, ½ cup	671
Carrots, frozen, cooked, ½ cup	607
Spinach, frozen, cooked, ½ cup	573
Spinach, canned, ½ cup	525
Sweet potato, canned, ½ cup	508
Collards, frozen, cooked, ½ cup	489
Kale, frozen, cooked, ½ cup	478
Mixed vegetables, canned, ½ cup	475
Spinach, fresh, cooked, ½ cup	472
Turnip greens, frozen, cooked, ½ cup	441
Instant cooked cereals, fortified, prepared, 1 packet	285–376
Various ready-to-eat cereals, added vitamin A, 1 oz.	180–376

Chunky vegetable soup, canned, 1 cup	290
Beet greens, cooked, ½ cup	276
Cantaloupe cubes, 1 cup	270
Winter squash, cooked, ½ cup	268
Mustard greens, cooked, ½ cup	221
Mixed vegetables, frozen, cooked, ½ cup	195
Red sweet pepper, cooked, ½ cup	186
Milk, fortified (fat-free, 1 percent, 2 percent), 1 cup	145
Apricot halves, canned, ½ cup	104
Egg, whole, large, cooked	85
Cheddar cheese, 1 oz.	75
Broccoli pieces, frozen, cooked, ½ cup	52
Margarine, regular, 1 tsp.	40
Apricot halves, 5	32
Broccoli, raw, 1 cup	27

Values based on USDA National Nutrient Database for Standard Reference, Release 18.

8. Calcium Content of Selected Foods

Adequate intake of calcium for individuals 9–18 years of age is 1,300 mg/day; at 19–50 years, 1,000 mg/day; more than 50 years, 1,200 mg/day.

Non-Dairy Food Sources	Calcium, mg	Dairy Food Sources	Calcium, mg
Fortified ready-to-eat cereals, various, 1 oz	236–1,043	Canned evaporated nonfat milk, 1 cup	742
Soy beverage, calcium fortified, 1 cup	368	Plain yogurt, low-fat (12 g protein/ 8 oz), 8-oz container	415
Sardines, Atlantic, in oil, drained, 3 oz	325	Fruit yogurt, low-fat (10 g protein/8 oz), 8-oz container	345
Pink salmon, canned, with bone, 3 oz	181	Ricotta cheese, part skim, ½ cup	335

(continued)

(continued)

Non-Dairy Food Sources	Calcium, mg	Dairy Food Sources	Calcium, mg
Collards, frozen, cooked, ½ cup	178	Fat-free (skim) milk, 1 cup	306
Rhubarb, frozen, cooked with sugar, ½ cup	174	1 percent low-fat milk, 1 cup	290
Tofu, firm, prepared with nigari[a], ¼ block	163	2 percent reduced fat milk 1 cup	285
Spinach, frozen, cooked, ½ cup	146	Buttermilk, low-fat, 1 cup	284
Soybeans, green, cooked, ½ cup	130	Chocolate milk, 1 cup	276
Oatmeal, plain and flavored, instant, fortified, 1 packet prepared	99–110	Whole milk, 1 cup	276
Ocean perch, Atlantic, cooked, 3 oz	116	Swiss cheese, 1 oz	224
Cowpeas, cooked, ½ cup	106	Provolone cheese, 1 oz	214
Kale, frozen, cooked, ½ cup	90	Mozzarella cheese, part-skim, 1 oz	207
Okra, frozen, cooked, ½ cup	88	Pasteurized process American cheese food, 1 oz	162
Soybeans, mature, cooked, ½ cup	88	Puddings, dry mix, instant, ½ cup	153
Clams, canned, 3 oz	78	Ice creams, vanilla, light, ½ cup	106
Blue crab, canned, 3 oz	86	Puddings, vanilla, ready-to-eat, ½ cup	99
Refried beans, canned, ½ cup	44	Ice creams, vanilla, ½ cup	84

[a] calcium sulfate and magnesium chloride

Values based on USDA National Nutrient Database for Standard Reference, Release 18.

9. Zinc Content of Selected Foods

The Recommended Dietary Allowance (RDA) for adults (19 years and older) is 8 mg/day for women and 11 mg/day for men. The Tolerable Upper Intake Level (UL) for adults is 40 mg/day. Adverse effects associated with chronic intake of supplemental zinc include decreased immune response, decrease in high-density lipoprotein (HDL) cholesterol, and reduced copper status. (National Academy of Sciences, 2000)

Food	Zinc, mg
Fortified ready-to-eat cereals, various, 1 cup	3–17
Beans, baked, canned, with pork and tomato sauce, 1 cup	13.9
Soup, oyster stew, canned, prepared with equal volume milk, 1 cup	10.3
Crab, Alaska king, cooked, moist heat, 3 oz	6.48
Beef, chuck, arm pot roast, separable lean and fat, trimmed to ⅛ ″ fat, choice, cooked, braised, 3 oz	5.84
Beef, ground, 80% lean meat/20% fat, cooked, 3 oz.	5.16
Ready-to-eat cereals, Cheerios, 1 cup	4.62
Lamb, domestic, shoulder, arm, separable lean and fat, trimmed to ¼ ″ fat, choice, cooked, 1 chop	3.81
Soup, black bean, canned, 1 cup	2.83
Chicken, leg (thigh and drumstick), broiled, without skin, 1 leg	2.72
Lobster, northern, cooked, moist heat, 3 oz	2.48
Wheat germ, toasted, plain, 2 tablespoons	2.35
Beans, navy, canned, 1 cup	2.02
Pork, loin, sirloin (chops) or ham, cooked, 3 oz	2.00
Yogurt, fruit, low fat, 10 grams protein per 8 oz., 1 cup	1.81
Turkey, fryer-roasters, breast, cooked, 3 oz	1.51
Chicken, broilers or fryers, breast, cooked, 1 cup diced	1.40
Peanut butter, smooth style, 2 tablespoons	0.93
Cheese, cheddar, 1 oz	0.88
Seeds, pumpkin and squash seeds, whole, roasted, ⅛ cup	0.82
Cheese, ricotta, part skim milk, ¼ cup	0.82
Peas, green, frozen, cooked, ½ cup	0.75
Bread, whole-wheat, 1 slice	0.54
Fish, haddock, cooked, dry heat, 3 oz	0.41
Corn, sweet, yellow, canned, whole kernel, ½ cup	0.32

Nutrient values from Agricultural Research Service (ARS) Nutrient Database for Standard Reference, Release 18

10. Iron Content of Selected Foods

Food sources of iron ranked by milligrams of iron per standard serving size. The Recommended Daily Allowance is 8 mg/d for men 19 years and older; 18 mg/d for females 19–50 years; and 8 mg/d for females 51 years and older.

Food, Standard Amount	Iron, mg
Clams, canned, drained, 3 oz	23.8
Fortified ready-to-eat cereals, various, ~ 1 oz	1.8–21.1
Fortified instant cooked cereals, various, 1 packet	4.9–8.1
Chili con carne with beans, canned entrée, 1 cup	5.8
Oysters, wild, cooked, moist heat, 6 medium	5.6
Soybeans, mature, cooked, ½ cup	4.4
Lentils, cooked, ½ cup	3.3
Spinach, cooked, ½ cup	3.2
Beef, chuck, blade roast, lean, cooked, 3 oz	3.1
Beef, round, bottom round, separable lean and fat, trimmed to ⅛ " fat, all grades, cooked, braised, 3 oz	2.38
Soybeans, green, cooked, ½ cup	2.3
Chicken, liver, all classes, cooked, simmered, 1 liver	2.3
Ground beef, 15% fat, cooked, 3 oz	2.2
Chicken, canned, meat only, with broth, 5 oz	2.2
Navy beans, cooked, ½ cup	2.3
Beef, ground, 80% lean meat / 20% fat, patty, cooked, 3 oz	2.1
Refried beans, canned, ½ cup	2.1
Lima beans, frozen, baby, cooked, ½ cup	1.8
Peas, edible-podded, boiled, ½ cup	1.6
Kidney beans, cooked, ½ cup	1.6
Beef, top sirloin, separable lean and fat, trimmed to ⅛ " fat, all grades, cooked, broiled, 3 oz	1.5
Tomato sauce, ½ cup	1.3
Seeds, sunflower seed kernels, dry roasted, with salt added, ¼ cup	1.2
Prune juice, ⅓ cup	1.0
Chicken, broilers or fryers, breast, meat only, cooked, roasted, ½ breast	0.9
Egg, whole, cooked, fried, 1 large	0.9
Collards, frozen, chopped, cooked, ½ cup	0.9
Pork, fresh, loin, center loin (chops), bone-in, separable lean and fat, cooked, broiled, 3 oz	0.7
Shrimp, cooked, breaded and fried, 6 large	0.6
Raisins, seedless, ¼ cup	0.6

Nutrient values from Agricultural Research Service (ARS) Nutrient Database for Standard Reference, Release 18

11. Exchange Lists for Meal Planning[1]

Foods are listed with their serving sizes, which are usually measured after cooking. When you begin, measuring the size of each serving will help you learn to "eyeball" correct serving sizes. The following chart shows the amount of nutrients in one serving from each list.

Groups/Lists	Carbohydrate (grams)	Protein (grams)	Fat (grams)	Calories
Carbohydrate Group				
Starch	15	3	0–1	80
Fruit	15	—	—	60
Milk				
Fat-free, low-fat	12	8	0–3	90
Reduced-fat	12	8	5	120
Whole	12	8	8	150
Other carbohydrates	15	varies	varies	varies
Nonstarchy vegetables	5	2	—	25
Meat and Meat Substitutes Group				
Very lean	—	7	0–1	35
Lean	—	7	3	55
Medium-fat	—	7	5	75
High-fat	—	7	8	100
Fat Group	—	—	5	45

Starch List

Cereals, grains, pasta, breads, crackers, snacks, starchy vegetables, and cooked beans, peas, and lentils are starches. In general, one starch is:

- ½ cup of cooked cereal, grain, or starchy vegetable
- ⅓ cup of cooked rice or pasta
- 1 oz of a bread product, such as 1 slice of bread
- ¾ to 1 oz of most snack foods (Some snack foods may also have added fat.)

[1]2003. American Dietetic Association. Used with permission.

■ **NUTRITION TIPS**
1. Most starch choices are good sources of B vitamins
2. Foods made from whole grains are good sources of fiber.

   - A serving from the bread list, on average, has 1 gram of fiber.
   - A serving from the cereals and grains list or the crackers and snacks list, on average, has 2 grams of fiber.
   - A serving from the starchy vegetables list, on average, has 3 grams of fiber.

3. Beans, peas, and lentils are good sources of protein and fiber.

   - A serving from the food group, on average, has 6 grams of fiber.

■ **SELECTION TIPS**
1. Choose starches made with little fat as often as you can.
2. Starchy vegetables prepared with fat count as one starch and one fat.
3. For many starchy foods (e.g., bagels, muffins, dinner rolls, buns), a general rule of thumb is 1 oz equals 1 carbohydrate serving. However, bagels or muffins range widely in size. Check the size you eat. Also, use the Nutrition Facts on food labels when available.
4. Beans, peas, and lentils are also found on the meat and meat substitutes list.
5. A waffle or pancake is about the size of a compact disc (CD) and about ¼ inch thick.
6. Because starches often swell in cooking, a small amount of uncooked starch will become a much larger amount of cooked food.
7. Most of the serving sizes are measured or weighed after cooking.
8. For specific information, check Nutrition Facts on the food label.

One starch exchange equals:
15 grams of carbohydrate
3 grams of protein
0–1 grams of fat
80 calories

Bread

Bagel, 4 oz	¼ (1 oz)
Bread, reduced-calorie	2 slices (1½ oz)
Bread, white, whole-wheat, pumpernickel, rye	1 slice (1 oz)
Bread sticks, crisp, 4 inch x ½ inch	4 (⅔ oz)
English muffin	½
Hot dog bun or hamburger bun	½ (1 oz)
Naan, 8 x 2 inch	¼
Pancake, 4 inch across, ¼ inch thick	1
Pita, 6 inch across	½
Roll, plain, small	1 (1 oz)
Raisin bread, unfrosted	1 slice (1 oz)
Tortilla, corn, 6 inch across	1
Tortilla, flour, 6 inch across	1
Tortilla flour, 10 inch across	⅓
Waffle, 4 inch square or across, reduced-fat	1

Cereals and Grains

Bran cereals	½ cup
Bulgur	½ cup
Cereals, cooked	½ cup
Cereals, unsweetened, ready-to-eat	¾ cup
Cornmeal (dry)	3 Tbsp
Couscous	⅓ cup
Flour (dry)	3 Tbsp
Granola, low-fat	¼ cup
Grape-Nuts	¼ cup
Grits	½ cup
Kasha	½ cup
Millet	⅓ cup
Muesli	¼ cup
Oats	½ cup
Pasta	⅓ cup
Puffed cereal	1½ cups
Rice, white or brown	⅓ cup
Shredded Wheat	½ cup
Sugar-frosted cereal	½ cup
Wheat germ	3 Tbsp

Starchy Vegetables

Baked beans	⅓ cup
Corn	½ cup

(continued)

Starchy Vegetables *(continued)*

Corn on cob, large	½ cob (5 oz)
Mixed vegetables with corn, peas, or pasta	1 cup
Peas, green	½ cup
Plantain	½ cup
Potato, boiled medium (3 oz)	½ cup or ½
Potato, baked with skin	¼ large (3 oz)
Potato, mashed	½ cup
Squash, winter (acorn, butternut, pumpkin)	1 cup
Yam, sweet potato, plain	½ cup

Crackers and Snacks

Animal crackers	8
Graham cracker, 2½ inch square	3
Matzoh	¾ oz
Melba toast	4 slices
Oyster crackers	20
Popcorn (popped, no fat added, or low-fat microwave)	3 cups
Pretzels	¾ oz
Rice cakes, 4 inch across	2
Saltine-type crackers	6
Snack chips, fat-free or baked (tortilla, potato)	15–20 (¾ oz)
Whole-wheat crackers, no fat added	2–5 (¾ oz)

Beans, Peas, and Lentils
(count as 1 starch exchange, plus 1 very lean meat exchange)

Beans and peas (garbanzo, pinto, kidney, white, split, black-eyed)	½ cup
Lima beans	⅔ cup
Lentils	½ cup
Miso*	3 Tbsp

Starchy Foods Prepared with Fat
(count as 1 starch exchange, plus 1 fat exchange)

Biscuit, 2½ inch across	1
Chow mein noodles	½ cup
Corn bread, 2 inch cube	1 (2 oz)
Crackers, round butter type	6
Croutons	1 cup
French-fried potatoes (oven-baked) (see also fast foods list)	1 cup (2 oz)
Granola	¼ cup
Hummus	⅓ cup
Muffin, 5 oz	⅕ (1 oz)
Popcorn, microwaved	3 cups
Sandwich crackers, cheese or peanut butter filling	3

Snack chips (potato, tortilla)	9–13 (¾ oz)
Stuffing, bread (prepared)	⅓ cup
Taco shell, 5 inch across	2
Waffle, 4 inch square or across	1
Whole-wheat crackers, fat added	4–7 (1 oz)

* = 400 mg or more sodium per exchange

Fruit List

Fresh, frozen, canned, and dried fruits and fruit juices are on this list. In general, one fruit exchange is:

- 1 small fresh fruit (4 oz)
- ½ cup of canned or fresh fruit or unsweetened fruit juice
- ¼ cup of dried fruit

■ NUTRITION TIPS

1. Fresh, frozen, and dried fruits have about 2 grams of fiber per choice. Fruit juices contain very little fiber.
2. Citrus fruits, berries, and melons are good sources of vitamin C.

■ SELECTION TIPS

1. Count ½ cup cranberries or rhubarb sweetened with sugar substitutes as free foods.
2. Read the Nutrition Facts on the food label. If one serving has more than 15 grams of carbohydrate, you will need to adjust the size of the serving you eat or drink.
3. Portion sizes for canned fruits are for the fruit and a small amount of juice.
4. Whole fruit is more filling than fruit juice and may be a better choice.
5. Food labels for fruits may contain the words "no sugar added" or "unsweetened." This means that no sucrose (table sugar) has been added.
6. Generally, fruit canned in extra light syrup has the same amount of carbohydrate per serving as the "no sugar added" or the juice pack. All canned fruits on the fruit list are based on one of these three types of pack.

One fruit exchange equals:
15 grams of carbohydrate
60 calories

The weight includes skin, core, seeds, and rind.

Fruit

Apple, unpeeled, small	1 (4 oz)
Applesauce, unsweetened	½ cup
Apples, dried	4 rings
Apricots, fresh	4 whole (5½ oz)
Apricots, dried	8 halves
Apricots, canned	½ cup
Banana, small	1 (4 oz)
Blackberries	¾ cup
Blueberries	¾ cup
Cantaloupe, small	⅓ melon (11 oz) or 1 cup cubes
Cherries, sweet, fresh	12 (3 oz)
Cherries, sweet, canned	½ cup
Dates	3
Figs, fresh	1½ large or 2 medium (3½ oz)
Figs, dried	1½
Fruit cocktail	½ cup
Grapefruit, large	½ (11 oz)
Grapefruit sections, canned	¾ cup
Grapes, small	17 (3 oz)
Honeydew melon	1 slice (10 oz) or 1 cup cubes
Kiwi	1 (3½ oz)
Mandarin oranges, canned	¾ cup
Mango, small	½ fruit (5½ oz or ½ cup)
Nectarine, small	1 (5 oz)
Orange, small	1 (6½ oz)
Papaya	½ fruit (8 oz) or 1 cup cubes
Peach, medium, fresh	1 (6 oz)
Peaches, canned	½ cup
Pear, large, fresh	½ (4 oz)
Pears, canned	½ cup
Pineapple, fresh	¾ cup
Pineapple, canned	½ cup
Plums, small	2 (5 oz)
Plums, canned	½ cup
Plums, dried (prunes)	3
Raisins	2 Tbsp
Raspberries	1 cup
Strawberries	1¼ cup whole berries
Tangerines, small	2 (8 oz)
Watermelon	1 slice (13½ oz) or 1¼ cup cubes

Fruit Juice, Unsweetened

Apple juice/cider	½ cup
Cranberry juice cocktail	⅓ cup
Cranberry juice cocktail, reduced-calorie	1 cup
Fruit juice blends, 100% juice	⅓ cup
Grape juice	⅓ cup
Grapefruit juice	½ cup
Orange juice	½ cup
Pineapple juice	½ cup
Prune juice	⅓ cup

Milk List

Different types of milk and milk products are on this list. Cheeses are on the meat and meat substitutes list and cream and other dairy fats are on the fat list. Based on the amount of fat they contain, milks are divided into fat-free/low-fat milk, reduced-fat milk, and whole milk. One choice of these includes:

	Carbohydrate (grams)	Protein (grams)	Fat (grams)	Calories
Fat-free/low-fat (½% or 1%)	12	8	0–3	90
Reduced-fat (2%)	12	8	5	120
Whole	12	8	8	150

■ **NUTRITION TIPS**
1. Milk and yogurt are good sources of calcium and protein. Check the Nutrition Facts on the food label.
2. The higher the fat content of milk and yogurt, the greater the amount of saturated fat and cholesterol. Choose lower-fat varieties.
3. For those who are lactose intolerant, look for lactose-reduced or lactose-free varieties of milk. Check the food label for the total amount of carbohydrate per serving.

■ **SELECTION TIPS**
1. 1 cup equals 8 fluid oz or ½ pint.
2. Look for chocolate milk, rice milk, frozen yogurt, and ice cream on the sweets, desserts, and other carbohydrates list.
3. Nondairy creamers are on the free foods list.
   One milk exchange equals:
   12 grams of carbohydrate
   8 grams of protein

Fat-Free and Low-Fat Milk	
(0–3 grams fat per serving)	
Fat-free milk	1 cup
½% milk	1 cup
1% milk	1 cup
Buttermilk, low-fat or fat-free	1 cup
Evaporated fat-free milk	½ cup
Fat-free dry milk	⅓ cup dry
Soy milk, low-fat or fat-free	1 cup
Yogurt, fat-free, flavored, sweetened with nonnutritive sweetener and fructose	6 oz
Yogurt, plain fat-free	6 oz
Reduced-Fat	
(5 grams fat per serving)	
2% milk	1 cup
Soy milk	1 cup
Sweet acidophilus milk	1 cup
Yogurt, plain low-fat	6 oz
Whole Milk	
(8 grams fat per serving)	
Whole milk	1 cup
Evaporated whole milk	½ cup
Goat's milk	1 cup
Kefir	1 cup
Yogurt, plain (made from whole milk)	8 oz

Sweets, Desserts, and Other Carbohydrates List

You can substitute food choices from this list for a starch, fruit, or milk choice on your meal plan. Some choices will also count as one or more fat choices.

■ NUTRITION TIPS

1. These foods can be substituted for other carbohydrate-containing foods in your meal plan, even though they contain added sugars or fat. However, they do not contain as many important vitamins and minerals as the choices on the starch, fruit, or milk list.
2. When choosing these foods, include foods from the other lists to eat balanced meals.

■ SELECTION TIPS

1. Because many of these foods are concentrated sources of carbohydrate and fat, saturated fat, and *trans* fat, the portion sizes are often very small.

2. Look for the words "hydrogenated" or "partially hydrogenated" on the ingredient label. The lower down on the list these words appear, the fewer *trans* fats there are.
3. Be sure to check the Nutrition Facts on the food label. It will be your most accurate source of information.
4. Many fat-free or reduced-fat products made with fat replacers contain carbohydrate. When eaten in large amounts, they may need to be counted. Talk with your dietitian to determine how to count these in your meal plan.
5. Look for fat-free salad dressings in smaller amounts on the free foods list.

One carbohydrate exchange equals:

15 grams of carbohydrate, or

1 starch, or 1 fruit, or 1 milk.

Food	Serving Size	Exchanges per Serving
Angel food cake, unfrosted	$1/12^{th}$ cake (about 2 oz)	2 carbohydrates
Brownie, small, unfrosted	2 inch square (about 1 oz)	1 carbohydrate, 1 fat
Cake, unfrosted	2 inch square (about 1 oz)	1 carbohydrate, 1 fat
Cake, frosted	2 inch square (about 2 oz)	2 carbohydrates, 1 fat
Cookie or sandwich cookie with creme filling	2 small (about ⅔ oz)	1 carbohydrate, 1 fat
Cookies, sugar-free	3 small or 1 large (¾ to 1 oz)	1 carbohydrate, 1–2 fats
Cranberry sauce, jellied	¼ cup	1½ carbohydrates
Cupcake, frosted	1 small (about 2 oz)	2 carbohydrates, 1 fat
Doughnut, plain cake	1 medium (1½ oz)	1½ carbohydrates, 2 fats
Doughnut, glazed	3¾ inch across (2 oz)	2 carbohydrates, 2 fats
Energy, sport, or breakfast bar	1 bar (1⅓ oz)	1½ carbohydrates, 0–1 fat
Energy, sport, or breakfast bar	1 bar (2 oz)	2 carbohydrates, 1 fat
Fruit cobbler	½ cup (3½ oz)	3 carbohydrates, 1 fat
Fruit juice bars, frozen, 100% juice	1 bar (3 oz)	1 carbohydrate
Fruit snacks, chewy (pureed fruit concentrate)	1 roll (¾ oz)	1 carbohydrate
Fruit spreads, 100% juice	1½ Tbsp	1 carbohydrate
Gelatin, regular	½ cup	1 carbohydrate
Gingersnaps	3	1 carbohydrate
Granola or snack bar, regular or low-fat	1 bar (1 oz)	1½ carbohydrates
Honey	1 Tbsp	1 carbohydrate

(continued)

(continued)

Food	Serving Size	Exchanges per Serving
Ice cream	½ cup	1 carbohydrate, 2 fats
Ice cream, light	½ cup	1 carbohydrate, 1 fat
Ice cream, low-fat	½ cup	1½ carbohydrates
Ice cream, fat-free, no sugar added	½ cup	1 carbohydrate
Jam or jelly, regular	1 Tbsp	1 carbohydrate
Milk, chocolate, whole	1 cup	2 carbohydrates, 1 fat
Pie, fruit, 2 crusts	⅙ of 8-inch commercially prepared pie	3 carbohydrates, 2 fats
Pie, pumpkin or custard	⅛ of 8-inch commercially prepared pie	2 carbohydrates, 2 fats
Pudding, regular (made with reduced-fat milk)	½ cup	2 carbohydrates
Pudding, sugar-free or sugar-free and fat-free (made with fat-free milk)	½ cup	1 carbohydrate
Reduced-calorie meal replacement (shake)	1 can (10–11 oz)	1½ carbohydrates, 0-1 fat
Rice milk, low-fat or fat-free, plain	1 cup	1 carbohydrate
Rice milk, low-fat, flavored	1 cup	1½ carbohydrates
Salad dressing, fat-free*	¼ cup	1 carbohydrate
Sherbet, sorbet	½ cup	2 carbohydrates
Spaghetti sauce or pasta sauce, canned*	½ cup	1 carbohydrate, 1 fat
Sports drinks	8 oz (1 cup)	1 carbohydrate
Sugar	1 Tbsp	1 carbohydrate
Sweet roll or Danish	1 (2½ oz)	2½ carbohydrates, 2 fats
Syrup, light	2 Tbsp	1 carbohydrate
Syrup, regular	1 Tbsp	1 carbohydrate
Syrup, regular	¼ cup	4 carbohydrates
Vanilla wafers	5	1 carbohydrate, 1 fat
Yogurt, frozen	½ cup	1 carbohydrate, 0–1 fat
Yogurt, frozen, fat-free	⅓ cup	1 carbohydrate
Yogurt, low-fat with fruit	1 cup	3 carbohydrates, 0–1 fat

* = 400 mg or more of sodium per exchange

Nonstarchy Vegetable List

Vegetables that contain small amounts of carbohydrate and calories are on this list. Vegetables contain important nutrients. Try to eat at least 2 or 3 vegetable choices each day. In general, one vegetable exchange is:

- $\frac{1}{2}$ cup of cooked vegetables or vegetable juice
- 1 cup of raw vegetables

If you eat 3 cups or more of raw vegetables or $1\frac{1}{2}$ cups of cooked vegetables at one meal, count them as 1 carbohydrate choice.

■ NUTRITION TIPS

1. Fresh and frozen vegetables have less added salt than canned vegetables. Drain and rinse canned vegetables if you want to remove some salt.
2. Choose more dark green and dark yellow vegetables, such as spinach, broccoli, romaine, carrots, chilies, and peppers.
3. Broccoli, brussels sprouts, cauliflower, greens, peppers, spinach, and tomatoes are good sources of vitamin C.
4. Vegetables contain 1 to 4 grams of fiber per serving.

■ SELECTION TIPS

1. A 1-cup portion of broccoli is a portion about the size of a light bulb.
2. Tomato sauce is different from spaghetti sauce, which is on the sweets, desserts, and other carbohydrates list.
3. Canned vegetables and juices are available without added salt.
4. Starchy vegetables such as corn, peas, winter squash, and potatoes that contain larger amounts of calories and carbohydrates are on the starch list.

   One vegetable exchange ($\frac{1}{2}$ cup cooked or 1 cup raw) equals:

   5 grams of carbohydrate

   2 grams of protein

   0 grams of fat

   25 calories

Artichoke	Mushrooms
Artichoke hearts	Okra
Asparagus	Onions
Beans (green, wax, Italian)	Pea pods
Bean sprouts	Peppers (all varieties)

(continued)

(continued)

Beets	Radishes
Broccoli	Salad greens (endive, escarole, lettuce, romaine, spinach)
Brussels sprouts	Sauerkraut*
Cabbage	Spinach
Carrots	Summer squash
Cauliflower	Tomato
Celery	Tomatoes, canned
Cucumber	Tomato sauce*
Eggplant	Tomato/vegetable juice*
Green onions or scallions	Turnips
Greens (collard, kale, mustard, turnip)	Water chestnuts
Kohlrabi	Watercress
Mixed vegetables (without corn, peas, or pasta)	Zucchini

* = 400 mg or more sodium per exchange

Meat and Meat Substitutes List

Meat and meat substitutes that contain both protein and fat are on this list. In general, one meat exchange is:

- 1 oz of meat, fish, poultry, or cheese
- ½ cup of beans, peas, or lentils

Based on the amount of fat they contain, meats are divided into very lean, lean, medium-fat, and high-fat lists. This is done so you can see which ones contain the least amount of fat. One ounce (one exchange) of each of these includes:

	Carbohydrate (grams)	Protein (grams)	Fat (grams)	Calories
Very lean	0	7	0–1	35
Lean	0	7	3	55
Medium-fat	0	7	5	75
High-fat	0	7	8	100

■ NUTRITION TIPS

1. Choose very lean and lean meat choices whenever possible. Items from the high-fat group are high in saturated fat, cholesterol, and calories and can raise blood cholesterol levels.
2. Beans, peas, and lentils are good sources of fiber, about 3 grams per serving.

3. Some processed meats, seafood, and soy products may contain carbohydrate when consumed in large amounts. Check the Nutrition Facts on the label to see if the amount is close to 15 grams. If so, count it as a carbohydrate choice as well as a meat choice.

■ **SELECTION TIPS**

1. Weigh meat after cooking and removing bones and fat. Four ounces of raw meat is equal to 3 oz of cooked meat. Some examples of meat portions are:

    - 1 oz cheese = 1 meat choice and is about the size of a 1-inch cube or 4 cubes the size of dice.
    - 2 oz meat = 2 meat choices, such as:
    - 1 small chicken leg or thigh
    - ½ cup cottage cheese or tuna
    - 3 oz meat = 3 meat choices and is about the size of a deck of cards, such as:
      1 medium pork chop
      1 small hamburger
      ½ of a whole chicken breast
      1 unbreaded fish fillet

2. Limit your choices from the high-fat group to three times per week or less.
3. Most grocery stores stock Select and Choice grades of meat. The Select grades of meat are the leanest. The Choice grades contain a moderate amount of fat, and Prime cuts of meat have the highest amount of fat.
4. "Hamburger" may contain added seasoning and fat, but ground beef does not.
5. Read labels to find products that are low in fat and cholesterol (5 grams of fat or less per serving).
6. Dried beans, peas, and lentils are also found on the starch list.
7. Peanut butter, in smaller amounts, is also found on the fat list.
8. Bacon, in smaller amounts, is also found on the fat list.
9. Don't be fooled by ground beef packages that say X% lean (e.g., 90% lean). This is the percentage of fat by weight, NOT the percentage of calories from fat. A 3.5 oz patty of this raw ground beef has about half of its calories from fat.
10. Meatless burgers are in the combination foods list (3 oz of soy based burger = ½ carbohydrate + 2 very lean meats; 3 oz of

vegetable and starch-based burger = 1 carbohydrate + 1 lean meat).

■ **MEAL PLANNING TIPS**
1. Bake, roast, broil, grill, poach, steam, or boil meat and fish rather than frying.
2. Place meat on a rack so the fat will drain off during cooking.
3. Use a nonstick spray and a nonstick pan to brown or fry foods.
4. Trim off visible fat or skin before or after cooking.
5. If you add flour, bread crumbs, coating mixes, fat, or marinades when cooking, ask your dietitian how to count it in your meal plan.

Very Lean Meat and Substitutes List

• One very lean meat exchange is equal to any one of the following items:

Poultry: Chicken or turkey (white meat, no skin), Cornish hen (no skin)	1 oz
Fish: Fresh or frozen cod, flounder, haddock, halibut, trout, lox (smoked salmon)*; tuna fresh or canned in water	1 oz
Shellfish: Clams, crab, lobster, scallops, shrimp, imitation shellfish	1 oz
Game: Duck or pheasant (no skin), venison, buffalo, ostrich	1 oz
Cheese with 1 gram of fat or less per ounce: Fat free or low-fat cottage cheese	¼ cup
Fat-free cheese	1 oz
Other: Processed sandwich with 1 gram of fat or less per ounce, such as deli thin, shaved meats, chipped beef*, turkey ham	1 oz
Egg whites	2
Egg substitutes	¼ cup
Hot dogs with 1 gram of fat or less per ounce*	1 oz
Kidney (high in cholesterol)	1 oz
Sausage with 1 gram of fat or less per ounce	1 oz

• Count the following items as one very lean meat and one starch exchange.

Beans, peas, lentils (cooked)	½ cup

* = 400 mg or more sodium per exchange

Lean Meat and Substitutes List

• One lean meat exchange is equal to any one of the following items:

Beef: USDA Select or Choice grades of lean beef trimmed of fat, such as round, sirloin, and flank steak; tenderloin; roast (rib, chuck, rump); steak (T-bone, porterhouse, cubed); ground round	1 oz
Pork: Lean pork, such as fresh ham; canned, cured, or boiled ham;	1 oz

Canadian bacon*; tenderloin, center loin chop

Lamb: Roast, chop, or leg	1 oz
Veal: Lean chop, roast	1 oz
Poultry: Chicken, turkey (dark meat, no skin), chicken (white-meat, with skin), domestic duck or goose (well-drained of fat, no skin)	1 oz
Fish: Herring (uncreamed or smoked)	1 oz
Oysters	6 medium
Salmon (fresh or canned), catfish	1 oz
Sardines (canned)	2 medium
Tuna (canned in oil, drained)	1 oz
Game: Goose (no skin), rabbit	1 oz
Cheese: 4½% fat free cottage cheese	¼ cup
Grated Parmesan	2 Tbsp
Cheeses with 3 grams of fat or less per ounce	1 oz
Other: Hot dogs with 3 grams of fat or less per ounce*	1 ½ oz
Processed sandwich meat with 3 grams of fat or less per ounce, such as turkey pastrami or kielbasa	1 oz
Liver, heart (high in cholesterol)	1 oz

* = 400 mg or more sodium per exchange

Medium-Fat Meat and Substitutes List

• One medium-fat meat exchange is equal to any one of the following items:

Beef: Most beef products fall into this category (ground beef, meatloaf, corned beef, short ribs, Prime grades of meat trimmed of fat, such as prime rib)	1 oz
Pork: Top loin, chop, Boston butt, cutlet	1 oz
Lamb: Rib roast, ground	1 oz
Veal: Cutlet (ground or cubed, unbreaded)	1 oz
Poultry: Chicken (dark meat, with skin), ground turkey or ground chicken, fried chicken (with skin)	1 oz
Fish: Any fried fish product	1 oz
Cheese with 5 grams or less fat per ounce: Feta	1 oz
Mozzarella	1 oz
Ricotta	¼ cup (2 oz)
Other: Egg (high in cholesterol, limit to 3 per week)	1
Sausage with 5 grams of fat or less per ounce	1 oz
Tempeh	¼ cup
Tofu	4 oz or ½ cup

High-Fat Meat and Substitutes List

Remember these items are high in saturated fat, cholesterol, and calories and may raise blood cholesterol levels if eaten on a regular basis.

- One high-fat meat exchange is equal to any one of the following items:

Pork: Spareribs, ground pork, pork sausage	1 oz
Cheese: All regular cheeses, such as American*, cheddar, Monterey Jack, Swiss	1 oz
Other: Processed sandwich meats with 8 grams of fat or less per ounce, such as bologna, pimento loaf, salami	1 oz
Sausage, such as bratwurst, Italian, knockwurst, Polish, smoked	1 oz
Hot dog (turkey or chicken)*	1 (10/lb)
Bacon	3 slices (20 slices/lb)
Peanut butter (contains unsaturated fat)	1 Tbsp

- Count the following items as 1 high-fat meat plus 1 fat exchange:

Hot dog (beef, pork, or combination)*	1 (10/lb)

---

* = 400 mg or more sodium per exchange

Fat List

Fats are divided into three groups, based on the main type of fat they contain: monounsaturated, polyunsaturated, and saturated. Monounsaturated and polyunsaturated fats in the foods we eat are linked with good health benefits. Saturated fats and fats called *trans* fatty acids (or *trans* unsaturated fatty acids) are linked with heart disease. In general, one fat exchange is:

- 1 teaspoon of regular margarine or vegetable oil
- 1 tablespoon of regular salad dressing

▪ NUTRITION TIPS

1. All fats are high in calories. Limit serving sizes for good nutrition and health.
2. Nuts and seeds contain small amounts of fiber, protein, and magnesium.
3. If blood pressure is a concern, choose fats in the unsalted form to help lower sodium intake, such as unsalted peanuts.

▪ SELECTION TIPS

1. Check the Nutrition Facts on food labels for serving sizes. One fat exchange is based on a serving size containing 5 grams of fat.
2. The Nutrition Facts on the food labels usually list total fat grams and saturated fat grams per serving. When most of the calories come from saturated fat, the food fits into the saturated fats list.

3. Occasionally the Nutrition Facts on food labels will list monoun-saturated and/or polyunsaturated fats in addition to total and satu-rated fats. If more than half the total is monounsaturated, the food fits into the monounsaturated fats list; if more than half is polyun-saturated, the food fits into the polyunsaturated fats list.

4. When selecting fats to use with your meal plan, consider replac-ing saturated fats with monounsaturated fats.

5. When selecting regular margarine, choose those with liquid veg-etable oil as the first ingredient. Soft margarines are not as satu-rated as stick margarines and are healthier choices.

6. Avoid foods on the fat list (such as margarines) listing hydro-genated or partially hydrogenated fat as the first ingredient be-cause these foods will contain higher amounts of *trans* fatty acids.

7. When selecting reduced-fat or lower-fat margarines, look for liq-uid vegetable oil as the second ingredient. Water is usually the first ingredient.

8. When used in smaller amounts, bacon and peanut butter are counted as fat choices. When used in larger amounts, they are counted as high-fat meat choices.

9. Fat-free salad dressings are on the sweets, desserts, and other car-bohydrates list and the free foods list.

10. See the free foods list for nondairy coffee creamers, whipped top-ping, and fat-free products, such as margarines, salad dressings, mayonnaise, sour cream, cream cheese, and nonstick cooking spray.

One fat exchange equals:

5 grams fat

45 calories

Monounsaturated Fats List

Avocado, medium	2 Tbsp (1 oz)
Oil (canola, olive, peanut)	1 tsp
Olives: ripe (black)	8 large
green, stuffed*	10 large
Nuts: almonds, cashews	6 nuts
mixed (50% peanuts)	6 nuts
peanuts	10 nuts
pecans	4 halves
Peanut butter, smooth or crunchy	½ Tbsp
Sesame seeds	1 Tbsp
Tahini or sesame paste	2 tsp

* = 400 mg or more sodium per exchange

Polyunsaturated Fats List

Margarine: stick, tub, or squeeze	1 tsp
lower-fat spread (30% to 50% vegetable oil)	1 Tbsp
Mayonnaise: regular	1 tsp
reduced-fat	1 Tbsp
Nuts: walnuts, English	4 halves
Oil (corn, safflower, soybean)	1 tsp
Salad dressing: regular*	1 Tbsp
reduced-fat	2 Tbsp
Miracle Whip Salad Dressing: regular	2 tsp
reduced-fat	1 Tbsp
Seeds: pumpkin, sunflower	1 Tbsp

Saturated Fats List

Bacon, cooked	1 slice (20 slices/lb)
Bacon, grease	1 tsp
Butter: stick	1 tsp
whipped	2 tsp
reduced-fat	1 Tbsp
Chitterlings, boiled	2 Tbsp (½ oz)
Coconut, sweetened, shredded	2 Tbsp
Coconut milk	1 Tbsp
Cream, half and half	2 Tbsp
Cream cheese: regular	1 Tbsp (½ oz)
reduced-fat	1 ½ Tbsp (¾ oz)
Fatback or salt pork*	Use a piece 1 inch x 1 inch x ¼ inch if you plan to eat the fatback cooked with vegetables. Use a piece 2 inch x 1 inch x ½ inch when eating only the vegetables with the fatback removed.
Shortening or lard	1 tsp
Sour cream: regular	2 Tbsp
reduced-fat	3 Tbsp

* = 400 mg or more sodium per exchange

Free Foods List

A *free food* is any food or drink that contains less than 20 calories and less than or equal to 5 grams of carbohydrate per serving. Foods with a serving size listed should be limited to 3 servings per day. Be sure to spread them out throughout the day. If you eat all 3 servings at one time, it could raise your blood glucose level. Foods listed without a serving size can be eaten whenever you like.

Fat-Free or Reduced-Fat Foods

Cream cheese, fat-free	1 Tbsp (½ oz)
Creamers, nondairy, liquid	1 Tbsp
Creamers, nondairy, powdered	2 tsp
Mayonnaise, fat-free	1 Tbsp
Mayonnaise, reduced-fat	1 tsp
Margarine spread, fat-free	4 Tbsp
Margarine spread, reduced fat	1 tsp
Miracle Whip, fat-free	1 Tbsp
Miracle Whip, reduced-fat	1 tsp
Nonstick cooking spray	
Salad dressing, fat-free, or low-fat	1 Tbsp
Salad dressing, fat-free, Italian	2 Tbsp
Sour cream, fat-free, reduced-fat	1 Tbsp
Whipped topping, regular	1 Tbsp
Whipped topping, light or fat-free	2 Tbsp

Sugar-Free Foods

Candy, hard, sugar-free	1 candy
Gelatin dessert, sugar-free	
Gelatin, unflavored	
Gum, sugar-free	
Jam or jelly, light	2 tsp

Sugar substitutes: alternatives, or replacements that are approved by the Food and Drug Administration (FDA) are safe to use. Common brand names include: Equal (aspartame), Splenda (sucralose), Sprinkle Sweet (saccharin), Sweet One (acesulfame K), Sweet-10 (saccharin), Sugar Twin (saccharin), Sweet 'N Low (saccharin)

Syrup, sugar-free	2 Tbsp

Drinks

Bouillon, broth, consommé*	
Bouillon or broth, low-sodium	
Carbonated or mineral water	
Club soda	
Cocoa powder, unsweetened	1 Tbsp
Coffee	
Diet soft drinks, sugar-free	
Drink mixes, sugar-free	
Tea	
Tonic water, sugar-free	

* = 400 mg or more sodium per exchange

Condiments

Catsup	1 Tbsp
Horseradish	
Lemon juice	
Lime juice	
Mustard	
Pickle relish	
Pickles, dill*	1½ medium
Pickles, sweet (bread and butter)	2 slices
Pickles, sweet (gherkin)	¾ oz
Salsa	¼ cup
Soy sauce, regular or light*	1 Tbsp
Taco sauce	1 Tbsp
Vinegar	
Yogurt	2 Tbsp

* = 400 mg or more of sodium per exchange

Seasonings

Flavoring extracts
Garlic
Herbs, fresh or dried
Pimento
Spices
Tabasco or hot pepper sauce
Wine, used in cooking
Worcestershire sauce

Note: Be careful with seasonings that contain sodium or are salts, such as garlic or celery salt and lemon pepper.

Combination Foods List

Many of the foods we eat are mixed together in various combinations. These combination foods do not fit into any one exchange list. Often it is hard to tell what is in a casserole dish or prepared food item. This is a list of exchanges for some typical combination foods. This list will help you fit these foods into your meal plan. Ask your dietitian for information about any other combination foods you would like to eat.

Food	Serving Size	Exchanges per Serving
Entrees		
Tuna noodle casserole, lasagna, spaghetti with meatballs, chili with beans, macaroni and cheese*	1 cup (8 oz)	2 carbohydrates, 2 medium-fat meats
Chow mein (without noodles or rice)*	2 cups (16 oz)	1 carbohydrate, 2 lean meats
Tuna or chicken salad	½ cup (3½ oz)	½ carbohydrate, 2 lean meats, 1 fat
Frozen entrees and meals		
Dinner-type meal*	generally 14–17 oz	3 carbohydrates, 3 medium-fat meats, 3 fats
Meatless burger, soy based	3 oz	½ carbohydrate, 2 lean meats
Meatless burger, vegetable and starch based	3 oz	1 carbohydrate, 1 lean meat
Pizza, cheese, thin crust*	¼ of 12 inch (4½–5 oz)	2 carbohydrates, 2 medium-fat meats
Pizza, meat topping, thin crust*	¼ of 12 inch (5 oz)	2 carbohydrates, 2 medium-fat meats, 1 ½ fats
Pot pie*	1 (7 oz)	2½ carbohydrates, 1 medium-fat meat, 3 fats
Entrée or meal with less than 340 calories*	about 8–11 oz	2–3 carbohydrates, 1–2 lean meats
Soups		
Bean*	1 cup	1 carbohydrate, 1 very lean meat
Cream (made with water)*	1 cup (8 oz)	1 carbohydrate, 1 fat
Instant*	6 oz prepared	1 carbohydrate
Instant with beans/lentils*	8 oz prepared	2½ carbohydrates, 1 very lean meat
Split pea (made with water)*	½ cup (4 oz)	1 carbohydrate
Tomato (made with water)*	1 cup (8 oz)	1 carbohydrate
Vegetable beef, chicken noodle, or other broth-type*	1 cup (8 oz)	1 carbohydrate

* = 400 mg or more sodium per exchange

Fast Foods List

Ask at your fast-food restaurant for nutrition information about your favorite fast foods or check web sites.

Food	Serving Size	Exchanges per Serving
Burrito*	1 (5–7 oz)	3 carbohydrates, 1 medium-fat meat, 1 fat
Chicken nuggets*	6	1 carbohydrate, 2 medium-fat meats, 1 fat
Chicken breast and wing, breaded and fried*	1 each	1 carbohydrate, 4 medium-fat meats, 2 fats
Chicken sandwich, grilled*	1	2 carbohydrates, 3 very lean meats
Chicken wings, hot*	6 (5 oz)	5 medium-fat meats, 1½ fats
Fish sandwich/tarter sauce*	1	3 carbohydrates, 1 medium-fat meat, 3 fats
French fries*	1 medium serving (5 oz)	4 carbohydrates, 4 fats
Hamburger, regular	1	2 carbohydrates, 2 medium-fat meats
Hamburger, large*	1	2 carbohydrates, 3 medium-fat meats, 1 fat
Hot dog with bun*	1	1 carbohydrate, 1 high-fat meat, 1 fat
Individual pan pizza*	1	5 carbohydrates, 3 medium-fat meats, 3 fats
Pizza, cheese, thin crust*	¼ of 12 inch (about 6 oz)	2½ carbohydrates, 2 medium-fat meats, 1½ fats
Pizza, meat, thin crust*	¼ of 12 inch (about 6 oz)	2½ carbohydrates, 2 medium-fat meats, 2 fats
Soft-serve cone	1 small (5 oz)	2½ carbohydrates, 1 fat
Submarine sandwich* (regular)	1 sub (6 inch)	3½ carbohydrates, 2 medium-fat meats, 1 fat
Submarine sandwich* (less than 6 grams fat)	1 sub (6 inch)	3 carbohydrates, 2 very lean meats
Taco, hard or soft shell*	1 (3–3½ oz)	1 carbohydrate, 1 medium-fat meat, 1 fat

* = 400 mg or more of sodium per exchange

12. Study Guide Suggested Responses

The following are suggested responses to Study Guide Questions in this book. Many questions have several acceptable answers. Responses comparable to those given here should be considered correct.

Chapter 1: Guidelines for Diet Planning

A. Consume a variety of foods within and among the basic food groups
   Control calorie intakes
   Be physically active daily
   Increase daily intakes of fruits and vegetables, whole grains, and low-fat milk and milk products
   Choose fats wisely for good health
   Choose carbohydrates wisely for good health
   Choose and prepare foods with little salt
   If you drink alcoholic beverages, do so in moderation
   Keep food safe to eat
B. Fruits: 1.5 cups
   Vegetables: 2.5 cups
   Grains: 6 oz-eq
   Meat & Beans: 5 oz-eq
   Milk: 3 cups
   Oils: 5 tsp
   How many discretionary calories are allowed? 195
C. Grains: dietary fiber, thiamin, riboflavin, niacin, folate, iron, magnesium, selenium
   Vegetables: potassium, dietary fiber, folate, vitamin A, vitamin E, vitamin C
   Fruits: potassium, dietary fiber, folate, vitamin C
   Meats & Beans: protein, niacin, thiamin, riboflavin, B-6, vitamin E, iron, zinc, magnesium
   Milk: calcium, potassium, vitamin D, protein
D. Every other day
E. See List in Chapter 1 or Appendix 7.
F. See List in Chapter 1 or Appendix 7.
G. Daily
H. See List in Chapter 1.
   See List in Chapter 1.

Chapter 2: Routine Diets

A. Economic, functional, physiological, psychosocial
B. Food stamps, home delivered meals, congregate meals, food pantries
C. See list of 22 in Chapter 2.
D. Use patterns to evaluate.
E. Iron, folate, zinc, protein, calcium
F. See list of 12 in Chapter 2.
G. Cut food into small pieces; remove seeds, skin, & bones. Cut round foods. Wait until 2 years of age to introduce peanut butter. Have child sit while eating, supervise meals.

Chapter 3: Consistency Altered Diets

A. Alterations in chewing and swallowing
B. Radiological physician, a swallowing therapist (speech language pathologist or occupational therapist), a dietitian, a nurse
C. See Chapter 3.
D. Thin, Nectar-like, Honey-like, Spoon-thick
E. Use patterns to evaluate.
F. Measure out desired number of servings.
   Measure the volume of the food after it has been pureed.
   Divide the total volume by the original number of portions.
   Reheat or chill following HACCP guidelines.

Chapter 4: Liquid Diets and Modifications

A. Preoperative preparation, postoperative care, acute inflammatory condition of the GI tract, acute stages of many illnesses, especially those with fever, conditions when it is necessary to minimize fecal material
B. Use Clear Liquid Diet Food for the Day table.
C. Use patterns to evaluate.
D. Soft-cooked or scrambled eggs; cottage cheese; baked (no skin), boiled, mashed, or creamed potatoes; refined cooked cereals; quick-type oatmeal; toasted white bread; soda crackers
E. Selection, administration, complications, information sources

Chapter 5: Diets for Weight Management

A. (1) 66%
   (2) 30.5%
   (3) Near $117 billion

B. Type 2 diabetes, cardiopulmonary disease, stroke, hypertension, gallbladder disease, osteoarthritis, sleep apnea, some forms of cancer

C. Diet therapy, physical activity, behavior therapy.

D. Use patterns to evaluate.

E. Use patterns to evaluate.

Chapter 6: Diets for Diabetes

A. Define/Differentiate the following

- Type 1 diabetes: auto-immune disease that affects the pancreas in a way that it does not release insulin.
- Type 2 diabetes: a disease that progressively results in the inability of the pancreas to function properly.
- Gestational diabetes: occurs only during pregnancy.

B. Diet, exercise, weight management

C. Maintaining as near normal blood glucose levels as possible; achieving optimal serum lipid levels; providing adequate energy to achieve & maintain a reasonable body weight in adults and to support growth during pregnancy & childhood; preventing & treating short & long term complications; improving overall health through optimal nutrition.

D. (1) Starches (2) Fruit and fruit juices (3) Milk & milk products (4) Sweets, desserts, and other carbohydrates

E. 15

F. Use patterns to evaluate.

G. Use patterns to evaluate.

H. Feeling shaky, sweaty, tired, hungry, crabby, confused, rapid heart rate, blurred vision or headaches, numbness or tingling in the mouth & lips; in severe cases, loss of consciousness.

I. See Treatment of Low Blood Sugar "Rule of 15" table; i.e. 12 animal crackers, ½ banana.

Chapter 7: Fat Restricted Diets

A. Diseases of the gallbladder, liver, or pancreas, disturbances in digestion or fat absorption, diet management of high blood cholesterol and other blood lipids

B. 40–50 grams of fat per day

C. Foods prepared with partially hydrogenated vegetable oils, commercially prepared fried foods, some margarines, fried foods served in restaurants.

D. The Cholesterol/Saturated Fat Restricted Diet limits cholesterol to less than 200 mg cholesterol, 25% to 35% of calories from fat.

E. See list of eight Diet Principles in Chapter 7.

F. Use Suggested Menu Plans to evaluate.

Chapter 8: Sodium Restricted Diets

A. 3,000–4,000 mg per day

B. Hypertension, edema

C. Use Food for the Day table for No Added Salt Diet.

D. 2,000 mg per day

E. Use Suggested Menu Plans to evaluate.

Chapter 9: Diets for Renal and Liver Disease

A. Liver, kidney

B. Registered dietitian

C. Eggs, dairy products, poultry, fish, meat

D. To ensure that protein is used for tissue growth & repair rather than for energy needs.

E. Protein, potassium, phosphorus

F. Pudding

G. Potassium

H. Use patterns to evaluate.

I. Use the Sample Meal Patterns table for the Protein and Electrolyte Controlled Diet.

Chapter 10: Fiber Modified Diets

A. Obesity, cardiovascular disease, type 2 diabetes, colonic diverticulosis, constipation

B. 25–30 grams

C. Abdominal discomfort, bloating, cramping, diarrhea

D. Constipation or impaction

E. Constipation, diverticular disease, colon cancer

F. Use High Fiber Diet Food for the Day table to evaluate.

Chapter 11: Other Modified Diets

A. Debilitating disease, surgery, healing of pressure ulcers, prevention of malnutrition in individuals with cognitive impairment, lack of appetite, or inability to eat normal portions of food

B. Calories, protein, minerals & vitamins

C. Use Outstanding Sources of Vitamin C listed in Chapter 1 under "Fruit Group."

D. Use Zinc Content of Selected Foods, Appendix 9.

E. Using half & half for cereal, extra butter or margarine at meals, super cereals, adding non-fat dry milk to prepared dishes. Multiple correct answers are possible.

F. Use Suggested Menu Plan for High Nutrient Diet to evaluate.

G. See list of eight Diet Principles for Finger Food Diet.

H. Vegan, Lacto-Vegetarian, Ovo-Lacto-Vegetarian, Semi-Vegetarian

I. Protein: plant proteins alone can provide enough amino acids when a variety of plant proteins are eaten and total caloric intakes are met.

Calcium: calcium intakes lower than recommended do not seem to cause health problems provided vitamin D intake or exposure to sunlight is adequate.

Iron: iron in plants is not as readily absorbed as iron in meats. To increase iron absorption, foods high in vitamin C should be offered at the same meal.

Vitamin B-12: only animal products contain B-12, vegans in particular need a reliable source of B-12, i.e. fortified cereals and soy beverages, brewer's yeast, vitamin supplements.

J. Food Allergy: abnormal response to a food triggered by the body's immune system

Food Intolerance: when eating a certain food triggers a negative physiological response, immune system is not affected

K. Milk, eggs, peanut allergy, tree nut allergy, fish & shellfish

L. Diminished production of lactase enzyme in the small intestine.

M. Commercial breads & baked goods, processed breakfast cereals, instant potatoes, soup & breakfast drink mixes, margarine, salad dressings, candies, snacks, mixes for pancakes, biscuits, cookies

N. Corn, rice, potato, soy, tapioca, bean, sorghum, amaranth, buckwheat, quinoa, teff, millet, Montina and nut flours

O. Modified food starch, hydrolyzed or texturized vegetable proteins, soy sauce, soy sauce solids, malt or malt flavoring

P. See list of six diet principles for Phenylalanine Restricted Diet.

Q. Avoid alcohol, quit smoking, avoid aspirin or NSAID medications, avoid foods which contribute to indigestion, reduce weight if obese, and avoid eating prior to bedtime.

Chapter 12: Dining Assistance/Special Needs

A. See Chapter 12, "Feeding Guidelines for Individuals with Dementia."

B. Individual

C. Individual

RESOURCES

References

1. Allred JB, Gallagher Allred CR, Bowers DF. 1990. Elevated blood cholesterol: a risk factor for heart disease that decreases with advanced age. *J AM Diet Assoc*. 90: 574–575.
2. American Diabetes Association Task Force. 2002. American Diabetes Association Position Statement: Evidence-based nutrition principles and recommendation for the treatment and preventing of diabetes and related complications. *J AM Diet Assoc*. 102: 109–118.
3. American Dietetic Association. 2000. *Manual of Clinical Dietetics*, 6th ed. Chicago: ADA.
4. ———. 2003. *Exchange Lists for Meal Planning*. Prepared by the American Dietetic Association and the American Diabetes Association. Chicago: ADA.
5. ———. 2002. *A Healthy Food Guide for People on Dialysis*. 2nd ed. Chicago: ADA.
6. ———. 2002. *A Healthy Food Guide for People with Kidney Diseases*. 2nd ed. Chicago: ADA.
7. ———. 2002. *National Dysphagia Diet Task Force*. Chicago: ADA.
8. ———. 2005. Position Paper of the American Dietetic Association: Liberalization of the diet prescription improves quality of life for older adults in long-term care. *J Am Diet Assoc*. Dec; 105 (12): 1955–65.
9. ———. 2005. Position Paper of the American Dietetic Association: Nutrition across the spectrum of aging. *J Am Diet Assoc*. Apr; 105 (4): 616–33.
10. ———. 1999. Position Paper of the American Dietetic Association: Medical nutrition therapy and pharmacotherapy. *J Am Diet Assoc*. Feb; 99 (2): 227–30. Review.

11. Baer MT, Farnan S, Mauer AM. 1990. Children with special health care needs. In: Sharbaugh C, ed. *Call to Action*. Washington DC: National Center for Education in Maternal and Child Health.
12. Blumberg J, Couris R. 1999. Pharmacology, nutrition and the elderly: Interactions and implications. In: Chernoff R, ed. *Geriatric Nutrition*. Gaithersburg, MD: Aspen Publishers Inc.: 342–365.
13. Chidester JC, Spangler AA. 1997. Fluid intake in the institutionalized elderly. *J Am Diet Assoc*. 1997 Jan; 97 (1): 23-8; quiz 29–30. Erratum in: *J Am Diet Assoc*. Jun; 97 (6): 584.
14. Clarke R, Refsum H, Birks J, Evans JG, Johnston C, Sherliker P, Ueland PM, Schneede J, McPartlin J, Nexo E, Scott JM. 2003. Screening for vitamin B-12 and folate deficiency in older persons. *Am J Clin Nutr*. May; 77 (5): 1241–7.
15. Dharmarajan TS, Adiga GU, Norkus EP. 2003. Vitamin B-12 deficiency. Recognizing subtle symptoms in older adults. *Geriatrics*. Mar; 58 (3): 30–4, 37–8.
16. Grabowski DC, Campbell CM, Ellis JE. 2005. Obesity and mortality in elderly nursing home residents. *J Gerontol A Biol Sci Med Sci*. Sept; 60 (9): 1184-9.
17. Heaney RP, Weaver CM. 2003. Calcium and vitamin D. *Endocrinol Metab Clin North Am*. Mar; 32 (1): 181–94, vii–viii.
18. Institute of Medicine, Food and Nutrition Board. 1997. *Dietary Reference Intakes for Calcium, Phosphorus, Magnesium, Vitamin D, and Fluoride*. Washington DC: National Academy Press.
19. _____. 1998. *Dietary Reference Intakes for Thiamin, Riboflavin, Niacin, Vitamin B6, Folate, Vitamin B12, Pantothenic Acid, Biotin, and Choline*. Washington, DC: National Academy Press.
20. _____. 2000. *Dietary Reference Intakes for Vitamin C, Vitamin E, Selenium, and Carotenoids*. Washington DC: National Academy Press.
21. _____. 2001. *Dietary Reference Intakes for Vitamin A, Vitamin K, Arsenic, Boron, Chromium, Copper, Iodine, Iron, Manganese, Molybdenum, Nickel, Silicon, Vanadium, and Zinc*. Washington, DC: National Academy of Sciences.
22. _____. 2002. *Dietary Reference Intakes for Energy, Carbohydrates, Fiber, Fat, Protein and Amino Acids (Macronutrients)*. Washington, DC: National Academy of Sciences.

23. Janssen I, Katzmarzyk P, Ross R. 2005. Body mass index is inversely related to mortality in older people after adjustment for waist circumference. *J Am Geriatr Soc.* 53 (12): 2112–2118.
24. Mahan LK, Ecott-Stump S. 2004. *Krause's Food, Nutrition and Diet Therapy,* 11th ed. Philadelphia, PA: Saunders.
25. Light KB, Hakkak R. 2003. Alcohol and Nutrition. *Handbook of Food-Drug Interactions.* 168–189.
26. Luchi RJ, Taffet GE, Teasdale TA. 1992. Congestive heart failure in the elderly. *J Am Geriatr Soc.* 40: 1109-1116.
27. *Merck Manual of Geriatrics.* 2001. Hoboken, NJ: Wiley, John & Sons, Inc.
28. McDonald RB, Ruhe RC. 2004. *The Progression from Physiological Aging to Disease: The Impact of Nutrition in Handbook of Clinical Nutrition and Aging* Ed. Bales CW, Ritchie CS. Totowa, NJ. Humana Press, Ch 3, 49–62.
29. Meyer C. 2004. The tea and toast syndrome: psychosocial aspects of congregate dining. *Generations.* xxvii (3): 92–94.
30. Modified Food Pyramid for Older Adults. 2003. Friedman School of Nutrition Science and Policy, Tufts University. http://nutrition.tufts.edu/consumer/pyramid.html (accessed November 1, 2005).
31. Niedert K, Dorner B. 2004. *Nutrition Care of the Older Adult: A Handbook for Dietetics Professionals Working Throughout the Continuum of Care.* 2nd ed. Chicago, IL: ADA.
32. Robinson GE, Leif BJ, eds. 2001. *Nutrition Management & Restorative Dining for Older Adults: Practical Interventions for Caregivers.* Chicago IL: ADA.
33. Schatz IJ, Masaki K, Yano K, Chen R, Rodriguez BL, Curb JD. 2001. Cholesterol and all-cause mortality in elderly people from the Honolulu Heart Program: a cohort study. *Lancet.* Aug 4; 358 (9279): 351–5.
34. Shiro-Harvey K. 2002. *National Renal Diet: Professional Guide.* 2nd ed. Chicago, IL: ADA.
35. Simons LA, Simons J, Friedlander Y, McCallum J. 2001. Cholesterol and other lipids predict coronary heart disease and ischaemic stroke in the elderly, but only in those below 70 years. *Atherosclerosis.* 159: 201–208.
36. Splett PL, Roth-Yousey LL, Vogelzang JL. 2003. Medical nutrition therapy for the prevention and treatment of unintentional weight loss in residential healthcare facilities. *J Am Diet Assoc.* Mar; 103 (3): 352–62.

37. Starling RD, Poehlman ET. 2000. Assessment of energy require-
    ments in elderly populations. *Eur J Clin Nutr*. Jun; 54 Suppl 3:
    S104–11.
38. Touger-Decker R, Mobley CC; American Dietetic Association.
    2003. Position of the American Dietetic Association: Oral health
    and nutrition. *J Am Diet Assoc*. May; 103(5): 615-25.
39. Tripp F. 1997. The use of dietary supplements in the elderly: cur-
    rent issues and recommendations. *J Am Diet Assoc*. Oct; 97 (10
    Suppl 2): S181–3.
40. Weinberg AD, Minaker KL. 1995. Dehydration. Evaluation and
    management in older adults. Council on Scientific Affairs,
    American Medical Association. *JAMA*. Nov 15; 274 (19):
    1552–6.
41. Wellman NS, Johnson MA. 2004. Translating the science of nu-
    trition into the art of healthy living. *Generations*. xxxviii (3):
    6–10.
42. Wilson MM, Morley JE. 2003. Invited review: Aging and energy
    balance. *J Appl Physiol*. Oct; 95 (4): 1728–36.
43. Yap HJ, Chen YC, Fang JT, Huang CC. 2002. Star fruit: A ne-
    glected but serious fruit intoxicant in chronic renal failure. *Dial
    & Transplant*. 31 (8): 564–7, 597.
44. United States Department of Health and Human Services,
    United States Department of Agriculture. 2005. *Dietary Guide-
    lines for Americans 2005*. www.health.gov/dietaryguidelines
    (accessed May 20 2005).

Internet Connections to Resources

American Diabetes Association: www.store.diabetes.org
American Dietetic Association: www.eatright.com/catalog
Blackwell Publishing: www.blackwellpublishing.com/food
Position Papers: www.eatright.org/public/index_7705.cfm
Dietary Guidelines for Americans, 2005: www.health.gov/
   dietaryguidelines/dga2005/document/
Evidence Analysis Library: www.adaevidencelibrary.com National
   Academy Press: www.NAP.edu
Nutrition Care Manual: www.nutritioncaremanual.org
USDA's MYPyramid Food Guidance System: www.mypyramid.gov
USDA National Nutrient Database for Standard Reference, Release 18
   Nutrient Lists: www.ars.usda.gov/services/docs.htm?docid=9673

INDEX

Entries followed by *f* indicate pages with figures.